T0226703

Diagnostics Stewardship in Molecular Microbiology: From at-home Testing to Next-Generation Sequencing

Editors

N. ESTHER BABADY
JENNIFER DIEN BARD

CLINICS IN LABORATORY MEDICINE

www.labmed.theclinics.com

Consulting Editor
MILENKO JOVAN TANASIJEVIC

March 2024 • Volume 44 • Number 1

ELSEVIER

1600 John F. Kennedy Boulevard • Suite 1800 • Philadelphia, Pennsylvania, 19103-2899

http://www.theclinics.com

CLINICS IN LABORATORY MEDICINE Volume 44, Number 1
March 2024 ISSN 0272-2712, ISBN-13: 978-0-443-12919-3

Editor: Taylor Hayes
Developmental Editor: Akshay Samson

Reprints. For copies of 100 or more, of articles in this publication, please contact the Commercial Reprints Department, Elsevier Inc., 360 Park Avenue South, New York, New York 10010-1710. Tel. 212-633-3874, Fax: 212-633-3820, E-mail: reprints@elsevier.com.

Clinics in Laboratory Medicine (ISSN 0272-2712) is published quarterly by Elsevier Inc., 360 Park Avenue South, New York, NY 10010-1710. Months of issue are March, June, September, and December. Business and Editorial offices: 1600 John F. Kennedy Blvd., Suite 1800, Philadelphia, PA 19103-2899. Periodicals postage paid at NewYork, NY and additional mailing offices. Subscription prices are $300.00 per year (US individuals), $100.00 per year (US students), $374.00 per year (Canadian individuals), $100.00 per year (Canadian students), $416.00 per year (international individuals), $185.00 (international students). For institutional access pricing please contact Customer Service via the contact information below. Foreign air speed delivery is included in all Clinics subscription prices. All prices are subject to change without notice. POSTMASTER: Send address changes to *Clinics in Laboratory Medicine*, Elsevier Health Sciences Division, Subscription Customer Service, 3251 Riverport Lane, Maryland Heights, MO 63043. **Customer Service: 1-800-654-2452 (US). From outside of the US and Canada, call 1-314-447-8871. Fax: 1-314-447-8029. E-mail: journalscustomerservice-usa@elsevier.com (for print support) or journalsonlinesupport-usa@elsevier.com (for online support).**

Clinics in Laboratory Medicine is covered in *EMBASE/Exerpta Medica, MEDLINE/PubMed (Index Medicus), Cinahl, Current Contents/Clinical Medicine, BIOSIS and ISI/BIOMED.*

Contributors

CONSULTING EDITOR

MILENKO JOVAN TANASIJEVIC, MD, MBA
Vice Chair for Clinical Pathology and Quality, Department of Pathology, Director of Clinical Laboratories, Brigham and Women's Hospital, Dana-Farber Cancer Institute, Associate Professor of Pathology, Harvard Medical School, Boston, Massachusetts

EDITORS

N. ESTHER BABADY, PhD, D(ABMM), FIDSA, FAAM
Chief, Clinical Microbiology Service, Attending Microbiologist and Professor, Department of Pathology and Laboratory Medicine, Department of Medicine (Infectious Disease Service), New York, New York

JENNIFER DIEN BARD, PhD, D(ABMM), FIDSA
Interim Chief, Laboratory Medicine, Director, Clinical Microbiology and Virology, Department of Pathology and Laboratory Medicine, Children's Hospital Los Angeles, Professor (Clinical Scholar) of Pathology, Keck School of Medicine, University of Southern California, Los Angeles, California

AUTHORS

RITU BANERJEE, MD, PhD
Professor, Division of Pediatric Infectious Diseases, Vanderbilt University Medical Center, Nashville, Tennessee

SUSAN M. BUTLER-WU, PhD, D(ABMM), FIDSA
Associate Professor, Department of Pathology, Keck School of Medicine of USC, University of Southern California, Los Angeles, California

DAN CHEN, PhD, D(ABCC)
Director of Clinical Chemistry, Department of Pathology, NYU Langone Health, New York, New York

AUGUSTO DULANTO CHIANG, MD
Assistant Professor, Division of Infectious Diseases, Vanderbilt University Medical Center, Nashville, Tennessee

CRISTINA COSTALES, MD
Assistant Director, Department of Pathology and Laboratory Medicine, Children's Hospital Los Angeles, Keck School of Medicine of USC, University of Southern California, Los Angeles, California

ARRYN CRANEY, PhD, D(ABMM)
Director, Center for Infectious Disease Diagnostics and Research, Diagnostic Medicine Institute, Geisinger Health System, Danville, Pennsylvania

KEVIN DEE, MD
Associate Professor, Division of Infectious Diseases, Vanderbilt University Medical Center, Nashville, Tennessee

JENNIFER DIEN BARD, PhD, D(ABMM), FIDSA
Interim Chief, Laboratory Medicine, Director, Clinical Microbiology and Virology, Department of Pathology and Laboratory Medicine, Children's Hospital Los Angeles, Professor (Clinical Scholar) of Pathology, Keck School of Medicine, University of Southern California, Los Angeles, California

CHRISTOPHER D. DOERN, PhD, D(ABMM)
Associate Professor, Department of Pathology, Virginia Commonwealth University Health System, Richmond, Virginia

DANIEL DULEK, MD
Assistant Professor, Division of Pediatric Infectious Diseases, Vanderbilt University Medical Center, Nashville, Tennessee

DAVID C. GASTON, MD, PhD
Assistant Professor, Department of Pathology, Microbiology, and Immunology, Vanderbilt University Medical Center, Nashville, Tennessee

ROMNEY M. HUMPHRIES, PhD, D(ABMM), FIDSA, FAAM
Professor, Department of Pathology, Microbiology, and Immunology, Vanderbilt University Medical Center, Nashville, Tennessee

CHELSEA KIDD, MD
Assistant Professor, Department of Pathology, Virginia Commonwealth University Health System, Richmond, Virginia

RACHAEL M. LIESMAN, PhD, D(ABMM)
Director, Clinical Microbiology and Molecular Diagnostics Pathology, Department of Pathology, Medical College of Wisconsin, Milwaukee, Wisconsin

JACKY LU, PhD
Post-Doctoral Fellow, Department of Pathology and Laboratory Medicine, Children's Hospital Los Angeles, Los Angeles, California

JOSE LUCAR, MD
Associate Professor, Division of Infectious Diseases, George Washington University School of Medicine and Health Sciences, Washington, DC

STEVE MILLER, MD, PhD
Chief Medical Officer, Delve Bio Inc, Department of Laboratory Medicine, University of California, San Francisco, San Francisco, California

ANISHA MISRA, PhD, D(ABMM)
Assistant Professor, Department of Laboratory Medicine, Cleveland Clinic, Robert J. Tomsich Pathology and Laboratory Medicine Institute, Cleveland, Ohio

HEBA H. MOSTAFA, MD, PhD, D(ABMM)
Associate Professor of Pathology, Director of Molecular Virology, Johns Hopkins School of Medicine, Baltimore, Maryland

CAITLIN OTTO, PhD, D(ABMM)
Director of Microbiology, Department of Pathology, NYU Langone Health, New York, New York

ELEANOR A. POWELL, PhD, D (ABMM)
Associate Professor, Department of Pathology and Laboratory Medicine, University of Cincinnati College of Medicine, Cincinnati, Ohio

REBECCA YEE, PhD, D(ABMM)
Assistant Professor, Department of Pathology, George Washington University School of Medicine and Health Sciences, Washington, DC

MEGHAN W. STAROLIS, PhD, HCLD (ABB)
National Science Director, Molecular Infectious Disease, Quest Diagnostics, Chantilly, Virginia

MARK A. ZAYDMAN, MD, PhD
Assistant Professor, Department of Pathology and Immunology, Washington University School of Medicine, St Louis, Missouri

Contents

CLINICS IN LABORATORY MEDICINE

FORTHCOMING ISSUES

June 2024
Molecular Pathology
Lauren Ritterhouse, *Editor*

September 2024
Hematology Laboratory in the Digital and Automation Age
Carlo Brugnara and Olga Pozdnyakova, *Editors*

December 2024
Laboratory Testing and Health Disparities
Dina N. Greene, *Editor*

RECENT ISSUES

December 2023
Myelodysplastic Syndromes
Alexa J. Siddon, *Editor*

September 2023
Advances in Clinical Cytometry
Christopher B. Hergott, *Editor*

June 2023
Point of Care Testing
Linoj Samuel, *Editor*

Preface

Nothing Basic About It: Guiding the Judicious Use of Diagnostic Tests

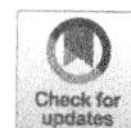

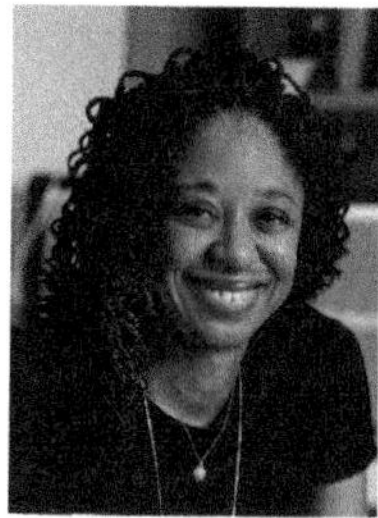

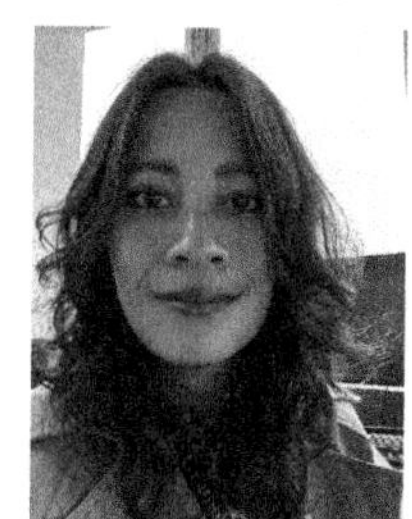

N. Esther Babady, PhD, D(ABMM), FIDSA, FAAM

Jennifer Dien Bard, PhD, D(ABMM), FIDSA

Editors

A lot has been written about the advent of molecular diagnostics and their impact on clinical care.[1,2] Without a doubt, since their introduction in clinical laboratories, molecular microbiology tests have resulted in better diagnostics and better patient care in a significantly shorter time to results. Innovation in enzyme chemistry and engineering has allowed for increased democratization of molecular testing to the point where testing is no longer limited to testing in high-complexity CLIA laboratories by highly trained medical laboratory scientists but available for use directly to the patient in the comfort of their home. An unbelievably powerful feat of human innovation. But as Uncle Ben told young Peter Parker in *Spider-Man*: "With great power comes great responsibility."[3] Guiding the judicious use of this powerful technology through diagnostic stewardship is a responsibility that places the medical microbiologist center stage.

This issue of *Clinics in Laboratory Medicine* not only includes topics that highlight the current state of molecular microbiology tests but also, more importantly, focuses on key concepts of diagnostic stewardship. As these molecular tests become simpler to both perform and interpret at the point-of-care, on one hand, and yet, more expensive and expansive in the amount and complexity of data produced on the other hand, it is imperative that medical microbiologists and other laboratorians use their expertise to lead the efforts to ensure that the right test is performed on the right patient at the right time.

In "Diagnostics Stewardship in Molecular Microbiology: From At-Home Testing to Next-Generation Sequencing," Dr Doern and Dr Kidds start by providing guidance on establishing a diagnostic stewardship committee with consideration on the committee membership as well as its tasks and responsibilities. Dr Susan Butler-Wu and

Clin Lab Med 44 (2024) xi–xiii
https://doi.org/10.1016/j.cll.2023.12.001
0272-2712/24/© 2023 Published by Elsevier Inc.

Dr Jacky Lu discuss the advent of at-home and CLIA-waived molecular microbiology and the best approaches for judicious use. Dr Otto and Dr Chen follow up by discussing the opportunities and challenges for establishing diagnostic stewardship programs for molecular testing performed in various point-of-care settings. As we move back into the laboratory setting, Dr Powell and Dr Misra remind us of one of the key tenets of Laboratory Medicine, "garbage in, garbage out," including special preanalytical considerations for molecular microbiology tests. Dr Yee and Dr Lucar focus on diagnostic stewardship for many of the commonly used syndromic panels, highlighting the fact that even simple tests require thoughtful implementation and use. Dr Starolis, Dr Zaydman, and Dr Liesman tackle the discussion of important but often neglected tools to optimize diagnostic stewardship, the laboratory, and clinical information systems.

As testing becomes more complex, the collaborative nature of diagnostic stewardship becomes even more critical. Dr Gaston and his colleagues from Vanderbilt University Medical Center, Dr Chiang, Dr Dulek, Dr Banerjee, Dr Humphries, and Dr Dee, provide an overview of diagnostic stewardship approaches for Next-Generation Sequencing (NGS), while Dr Costales and Dr Dien Bard discuss the critical role of the medical microbiologist in the implementation and interpretation of NGS tests. Dr Mostafa reminds us that while currently available molecular microbiology tests are not tests of infectiousness and shouldn't be used as such, to date, no other currently available methods exist for that purpose, and this remains a significant gap in testing. Dr Miller and Dr Craney wrap up the series by reminding us, not only of the central role of the medical microbiologist in diagnostic stewardship as new testing methodologies emerge but also of their responsibility in staying up-to-date with the scientific and technical bases underlying these tests.

We would like to thank all the amazing authors for their time and thoughtful contributions to this series. We believe that the readers will find the information useful and practical as they work on implementing diagnostic stewardship of molecular microbiology tests in their practice.

N. Esther Babady, PhD, D(ABMM), FIDSA, FAAM
Clinical Microbiology Service
Department of Pathology and
Laboratory Medicine

Department of Medicine
Memorial Sloan Kettering Cancer Center
New York, NY, USA

Jennifer Dien Bard, PhD, D(ABMM), FIDSA
Laboratory Medicine
Clinical Microbiology and Virology
Department of Pathology and Laboratory Medicine
Children's Hospital of Los Angeles
Keck School of Medicine
University of Southern California
Los Angeles, CA, USA

E-mail addresses:
babadyn@mskcc.org (N.E. Babady)
jdienbard@chla.usc.edu (J. Dien Bard)

REFERENCES

1. Fairfax MR, Salimnia H. Diagnostic molecular microbiology: a 2013 snapshot. Clin Lab Med 2013;33(4):787–803. https://doi.org/10.1016/j.cll.2013.08.003.
2. Highsmith WE Jr. Series, Molecular and Translational Medicine. Series, Molecular and Translational Medicine. New York, NY: Humana Press; 2014. https://doi.org/10.1007/978-1-4614-8127-0.
3. Lee S. Amazing adult fantasy #15. Available at: https://www.marvel.com/comics/series/13532/spider-man_with_great_power_comes_great_responsibility_2010_-_2011. Accessed October 21, 2023.

Taking Center Stage

Clinical Laboratory Leading Diagnostic Stewardship Efforts

Christopher D. Doern, PhD*, Chelsea Kidd, MD

KEYWORDS

• Stewardship • Utilization • Reference laboratory • Prior authorization
• Miscellaneous testing • Laboratory formulary

KEY POINTS

- Membership of a diagnostic stewardship committee should be multidisciplinary and include organization leaders who can support the committee's interventions.
- Minimizing utilization of "miscellaneous test" orders is essential to controlling referral laboratory testing.
- Establishing a laboratory test formulary process can help to control increasing utilization of reference testing.
- Direct-to-provider testing (testing that is sent without laboratory involvement) poses a serious compliance risk for organizations and is difficult to assess and control.

INTRODUCTION

The concept of diagnostic stewardship is quickly becoming a high priority for many institutions. Although diagnostic stewardship can mean many things and will almost certainly take different forms depending on an institution's needs, at its core, there are several principles that govern how it will be implemented. First, the goal of diagnostic stewardship is to ensure the appropriate usage of laboratory testing. There is a growing body of evidence suggesting that there is tremendous waste and overutilization of testing.[1] Factors contributing to this waste will be discussed in this review but the consequences are unnecessary cost, diagnostic confusion, and wasteful utilization of limited resources such as medical technologist time. Second, the complexities of referral laboratory testing, and all the different iterations, put institutions at risk of breaching patient confidentiality and being found in noncompliance with federal regulations. As will be discussed in this review, there are several pitfalls and challenges

Department of Pathology, Virginia Commonwealth University Health System, 403 North 13th Street, Richmond, VA 23298, USA
* Corresponding author.
E-mail address: christopher.doern@vcuhealth.org

Clin Lab Med 44 (2024) 1–12
https://doi.org/10.1016/j.cll.2023.10.004

with managing referral laboratory testing, many of which may not be obvious to the laboratory because they are handled independently of the routine referral laboratory process. These processes especially put institutions at great risk of financial loss and compliance violations.

This review should address issues faced by institutions, which are in the planning stages of forming diagnostic stewardship committees (DSCs), sometimes referred to as laboratory utilization committees, as well as those who have existing programs. Unfortunately, scientific evidence showing what should be done to start an effective diagnostic stewardship effort is sparing. As a result, much of this review will be based on personal experience and expert opinion. Where possible we will cite federal regulation and peer reviewed data but we will also lean on our own experiences and unpublished data.

Although many medical professionals who are involved in diagnostic stewardship care most about improving patient care, the dominant issue posed to DSCs is cost control. It is well recognized that one of the largest expenses for a laboratory operation is testing that is sent to external laboratories, sometimes referred to as reference laboratories. Due to the many challenges posed by this reference testing, it is prone to abuse and misunderstanding. As a result, it is an area of focus for most diagnostic stewardship efforts and newly formed programs will typically start in this area. In reviewing our own experiences, initial investigations into utilization of referral laboratory testing revealed several possible interventions, some of them easy wins, whereas others were much more challenging. The primary focus of this article will be to outline the efforts one might consider in controlling referral laboratory testing. There are several other reviews that have focused on elements of diagnostic stewardship, which more directly affect and improve patient care such as partnering with antimicrobial stewardship programs as well as the benefits of adopting rapid diagnostic technologies. These will not be discussed in this review, and the readers are referred to the following references.[2,3]

COMPONENTS OF DIAGNOSTIC STEWARDSHIP

The following sections will discuss the various components of diagnostic stewardship, including the makeup of a DSC, the specifics of analyzing referral laboratory testing, as well as some of the challenges one might encounter when developing their program. The following discussion is intended to be broadly applicable; however, some suggestions about specific tests and strategies will be included at the conclusion of this article.

Building of a Diagnostic Stewardship Committee

The foundation of a DSC is its members. Having gone through several different attempts to establish a robust and effective DSC, we have found that an essential element is support from the highest levels of the institution, including the chief medical officer as well as the chief operating officer and the chief executive officer. The support of these individuals as well as other hospital leaders is critical to maximizing the committee's effect. In the absence of this kind of support, the committee will often fail to implement the changes it deems necessary; this is especially true for those interventions that may be contentious and unpopular. Although these individuals do not necessarily have to be on the committee or participate actively, it is important to garner their support and even more effective if they are actively involved.

The membership of most committees will rely heavily on Pathology and Laboratory Medicine because they are typically the most invested group in these efforts.

However, external members are essential and add credibility and valuable insight into the committee's work. Some key groups that should be considered are the following: representatives from bone marrow transplant, solid organ transplant, genetics, neurology, pediatrics, internal medicine (especially infectious diseases), as well as emergency medicine. These are just a few suggestions of groups, which are important users of laboratory testing and will have valuable insight into how laboratory testing is used by their specialties as well as assist in managing changes in practice.

As with any committee, it is important to have individuals with primary responsibilities for ensuring that the committee's work moves along and does not become stagnant. It is recommended that at least 1 or 2 committee chairs be designated. The chair(s) can be from outside of the Department of Pathology and Laboratory Medicine; however, we have found that diagnostic stewardship work requires a detailed knowledge of the laboratory processes and access to laboratory data, making a chair from the Department of Pathology and Laboratory Medicine most effective. The disadvantage of this approach is that it can lead to the perception that the diagnostic stewardship activities are biased toward the needs of Pathology and Laboratory Medicine and do not necessarily consider the impacts on patient care and the needs of other departments. To be clear, these are perceptions but they may diminish provider buy-in.

Reference Laboratory Testing

Reference laboratory testing, in other words, testing that is performed at an external laboratory, is typically high volume and one of the largest expenditures for the Department of Pathology and Laboratory Medicine. For reasons that will be discussed in greater detail in later discussion, these expenditures are often not offset by reimbursement. To put this in perspective, a 1000-bed hospital system might send out close to 10,000 referral laboratory tests per year and spend well into the millions of dollars. There is evidence that the volume and cost of referral laboratory testing is increasing every year.[4] This is particularly challenging because the section of the laboratory tasked with managing send out tests is usually small and historically struggles to maintain full staffing. Staff in this area of the laboratory are not only responsible for packaging and sending specimens but also for answering questions, troubleshooting problems, resolving order discrepancies, and finally, ensuring that results are entered into the medical record.

With that said, there are several advantages to using referral laboratory testing. First, these laboratories can often achieve an economy of scale and offer testing for relatively inexpensive prices. Second, these laboratories can centralize hard-to-find expertise and make it easier to maintain competency. This is particularly useful for the performance of esoteric testing and testing for conditions that are not common.

The disadvantages of referral laboratory testing are that it can delay results compared with in-house testing. Delays are inevitable because specimens are sent to an external facility; however, delays may also result from challenges in entering patient results into the medical record. Most major reference laboratories will have the ability to establish interfaces with institutions so that results transfer directly into the patient's medical record. For smaller or rarely used reference laboratories, results are often not interfaced and must be entered manually. This can be a slow and error prone process.

Related to the activities of a DSC, reference laboratory testing poses unique challenges and opportunities. The most obvious opportunity is cost reduction by eliminating unnecessary testing. For a variety of reasons, reference laboratory testing is prone to abuse. The most nefarious cause of inappropriate use is due to direct-to-provider marketing by laboratories with questionable practices and offer esoteric testing that is of uncertain clinical utility. Often, these commercial laboratories offer testing, which is not reimbursable and/or may be coded incorrectly such that insurers will not pay for it. Therefore, it is essential that institutions verify the legitimacy of a laboratory and ideally, establish contracts with each of them. This can be particularly challenging because contracting processes are time-consuming and frequently take extended periods. There are significant compliance risks in sending testing to laboratories for which contracts have not been established. In these cases, the laboratory would be sharing patient information with unvetted entities, which may violate a patient's privacy. For these reasons, one goal of DSCs is to limit the number of reference laboratories that are used by an institution. The following sections discuss the various mechanisms by which a DSC might approach controlling reference laboratory testing.

Identifying Opportunities for Intervention

DSCs will find themselves with an abundance of opportunities for intervention. At the beginning of the efforts, although it can seem overwhelming, a good place to start is simply with a list of referral laboratory tests and the volumes of those tests. Depending on the goals of the program, it may also be useful to get the expenditures for each test, which can help prioritize intervention efforts. In general, laboratories will find that their most expensive send out tests come in 1 of 2 categories: either they are high volume but low-cost tests or they are lower volume but very expensive tests. Without exception, the latter category will include genetic testing for various conditions. A thorough discussion about the nuances of genetic testing is outside the scope of this review but it is important to recognize that these tests represent an area where stewardship can optimize patient care and physician understanding while also controlling cost. There are many different options and providers may have preferences for which laboratory a genetic test is sent to. DSCs will need to make sure providers are engaged to understand their preferences while also explaining the importance of standardizing testing for a given condition. It will not be uncommon for stewardship programs to encounter providers within the same practice that have different preferences for the same test. It has been our experience that trying to accommodate these individual preferences is untenable and quickly becomes too complicated for the laboratory to manage. Establishing a one test, one laboratory approach is essential for a successful stewardship program. Ideally, DSC's membership will include a genetics counselor to assist in managing the complexities of genetic testing.

Regarding high-volume testing, there are several potential issues that can be assessed to determine whether intervention is necessary. Often, high-volume tests will be subject to some amount of unnecessary ordering, which can be due to provider misunderstanding of the utility of the test and/or the frequency with which a test should be ordered. Unnecessary repeat or duplicate testing is particularly problematic for tests that may be trended to follow a disease condition or a response to therapy. Criteria may be used to define the frequency with which a test should be repeated, if at all. Some tests should only be done once in a lifetime, some tests may be trended, whereas others may be unintentionally repeated because the provider was unaware it had already been ordered. This is especially problematic for testing, which does not have a formal order built in a hospital's ordering system. This issue is discussed in greater detail in the "Miscellaneous Test Orders" section. Regardless of how a program wishes to limit repeat testing, it is recommended that their medical record system be used to enforce restrictions wherever possible. We have had excellent success in using a feature that notifies the provider of the fact that they are ordering a duplicate test while also presenting them with the previous test result. The immediate gratification of having a result presented without asking the provider to search through the medical record system has been well received and helped to build the credibility of the DSC. Regarding referral laboratory testing specifically, DSCs may also consider implementing a blanket restriction such that repeat testing cannot be performed before completion of the original result. We have found that a significant percentage of send out tests are repeated within hours of the original order, suggesting that the provider was simply unaware of the original order. This not only reduces expense but also spares the patient from having duplicate specimens collected and ultimately eliminates diagnostic confusion when duplicate tests return discrepant results.

Another method, which can identify inappropriate testing, is to look at the utilization of tests with a specific indication. For example, tests for invasive fungal disease, such as galactomannan and β-D-glucan, should only be used in immunocompromised patients who are at elevated risk for these kinds of infections.[5] If laboratories observe utilization by providers who do not care for immunocompromised patients, there might be an opportunity for intervention. Incorrect utilization also occurs when multiple tests are available for the diagnosis of the same condition. The diagnosis of Lyme disease, *Helicobacter pylori*, human immunodeficiency virus, and many other conditions all present a multitude of test modalities, which can be confusing to the ordering provider. A specific example from our own institution was the utilization of testosterone testing. We observed equal utilization of free testosterone as well as total testosterone. Free testosterone was a more expensive test that should not be used except in specific circumstances, whereas total testosterone was the more appropriate (and cheaper) test in most cases. By identifying the unusual ordering pattern, we were able to explore interventions and correct the misuse of free testosterone. Ultimately, it was determined that the incorrect ordering was a product of a provider misunderstanding of the indications for the 2 tests and a lack of awareness of the cost difference. Although it could not be proven, we also suspected that because the system presented free testosterone above total testosterone in the list of options, drove some of the inappropriate use. Through presenting the costs of each test and providing some limited guidance, we were able to drastically shift utilization.

Finally, talking to providers is an excellent way to identify laboratory utilization practices that may need to be addressed. Engaging providers in this way not only yields useful insights but will also start to build a collaborative and trusting relationship with the DSC.

Miscellaneous Test Orders

One challenge faced by all laboratories is the need to order tests that have not been built as official orders in the hospital's medical record system. There is an increasing array of esoteric laboratory tests such that it is impossible to have all built as orderable. Nor would that be useful because it would lead to an overwhelming number of options from which providers would have to choose. The solution to this problem is a generic order, often referred to as a "miscellaneous order" that allows the provider to enter the test they would want to order. Although this is a necessary feature, it poses significant problems from a utilization standpoint. First, it is difficult to standardize testing should a given test need to be ordered more than once. It is not uncommon for different providers to use the miscellaneous order to send the same test to 2 different laboratories. With inherent laboratory-to-laboratory performance variability, this practice can lead to inconsistency in results. Second, it is difficult for providers to know whether a test has been previously ordered for a patient, which may contribute to unintentional repeat testing. Third, it is difficult to ensure that tests are properly built and reimbursed if they are not officially orderable with all the appropriate coding that payers often require. In these cases, the referring laboratory will have to eat the cost of the test.

Fourth, the workflow around sending out a miscellaneous test is more difficult than an orderable test. Laboratory staff must ensure the accuracy of the information provided and whether a test can be performed at the requested laboratory. On receiving the laboratory results, the staff must manually enter the results into the medical record, which may require scanning of physical documents. Fifth, depending on how the miscellaneous test is displayed in the medical record, it may be very difficult for providers to find the results and act on them. Sixth, if the order a provider is looking for is not easily found in their search, they may assume it is not orderable and resort to the miscellaneous test option. Finally, physicians may request that testing be done at a laboratory with which there is no established relationship. This brings into question some of the significant compliance issues discussed above as well as challenges in billing and reimbursement.

It is in the laboratory's best interest to limit the amount of miscellaneous testing that is ordered for all the reasons discussed above. Although it is unlikely that the need for this generic order will ever be eliminated, the first step toward addressing the issue is to identify where miscellaneous tests are being ordered. Most institutions will have 1 or 2 primary major reference laboratories with which there is an established contract and often an interface for results to crossover into the medical record. This is an excellent place to look for miscellaneous tests. These major reference laboratories can provide lists of miscellaneous tests that have been sent to them which can make it easy to determine their volume and whether they should be built as orders. At our institution, we are attempting to minimize the need for a miscellaneous order and are building all tests that have been sent to a major reference laboratory as miscellaneous 2 or more times in the past year. Interestingly, we found that more than 60% of the miscellaneous tests we sent last year were to major reference laboratories. Thus, building these orders are "easy wins" because a contract and an interface are already established.

A more challenging task is to reduce the number of miscellaneous tests that are sent to smaller laboratories, especially if those laboratories do not have contracts with the institution. In contrast to miscellaneous orders sent to major reference laboratories, it is difficult to compile the usage data for these smaller laboratories. In our institution, the miscellaneous test order is a free text entry making it a manual process to pull reports to assess utilization.

Reviewing and building orders will be an ongoing effort for the DSC. In our institution, we have encountered an unexpected challenge in educating providers that an order no longer needs to be placed as miscellaneous. Providers may also have saved miscellaneous orders as "favorites" making it difficult to change provider ordering practice. Removing miscellaneous tests from favorite lists is a manual process, which requires information technology (IT) staff intervention and direct notification of providers. Ultimately, the goal of the DSC should be to reduce miscellaneous test volume so that individual orders can be reviewed and approved by the laboratory.

Creating a Laboratory Test Formulary

For all the reasons discussed earlier, an institution may attempt to eliminate or reduce the usage of the miscellaneous order and in its place, create a laboratory test formulary (LTF). Similar in concept to the Pharmacy and Therapeutics (P and T) committee, the goal of the LTF is to create a process by which tests can be reviewed and approved before implementation. To effectively implement an LTF approval process, the DSC must first minimize dependence on miscellaneous test ordering such that those can be reviewed and approved daily. An out-of-control miscellaneous testing process will allow providers to circumvent the LTF process by using the miscellaneous order. The following is a discussion of our DSC's process for reviewing and approving tests for our LTF.

Clinicians interested in adding a new test to the LTF are directed to contact the co-chairs of the DSC through a formal email address. In the early stages, many of the LTF requests come through forwarded email threads from groups who are unaware of the LTF process and have reached out to IT to request a new order build in our medical record system, or to purchasing, who manages collection kit orders. The understanding by these departments that approval by the DSC is required has been essential in proper review of new testing. It is hoped that over time the LTF will establish the same institutional presence as the P and T committee.

Individuals requesting a new test are provided with a submission form, which is reviewed by the cochairs. If the submission passes a preliminary cochair review, the submitter is invited to present their test request to the DSC. A short power-point template is provided to assist the requestor in formatting a brief 10-minute presentation to the committee. All materials are circulated and reviewed by the committee members in advance of the meeting, which occurs monthly. Following the presentation, there is a period of questioning and if possible, a vote to approve or deny the requested test. Often, outstanding questions cannot be resolved in the meeting, and a vote is delayed until those questions can be answered.

Regarding the decision to approve a test, the DSC makes that determination based solely on the clinical utility of the test. This is the first step in a long process of adding the test to the laboratory formulary. After approval by the committee, additional meetings between Pathology, billing, and IT occur to create a contract with any new laboratories and build the test into the medical record system with proper coding, prior authorization (as needed), and test restrictions. This can take a significant amount of time, and informing the individual who requested the test of the entire process is helpful to set expectations and assist with planning.

By building current miscellaneous tests and creating a process to handle new test requests, removal of the miscellaneous test order is theoretically possible. It is acknowledged that there will always be the need for an urgent test to be performed as miscellaneous. To address this need, a miscellaneous test "request" will be put into place to manage the rare situations of urgent testing needed, which is not built in the formulary; these orders will be reviewed in a timely manner by a designee of the DSC.

Prior Authorization

Prior authorization is the process of obtaining approval from payers before performing a test. For DSCs focused on cost control, this is an important issue to address because failing to obtain approval can lead to financial loss for the institution. Fortunately, a recent publication that reviewed prior authorizations pursued for pediatric genetic testing found high approval rates, although public payers were more likely than private insurers to approve testing (85% vs 70%).[6] Although that is good news, the mechanism by which one obtains prior authorization can be difficult.

Electronic medical record systems are not set up to facilitate obtaining prior authorization. Under normal circumstances, a test is ordered, a specimen is collected, sent to the laboratory, and the test is performed. Billing and reimbursement take place after testing is complete. This process does not work if prior authorization is required because approval must be obtained before the test is performed and ideally before the specimen is collected. One solution is to create a test "request" rather than a collectible order. This request triggers the prior authorization process, and if approved, a formal order can be placed. For this process to work, the laboratory and the provider must know what tests require prior authorization so that they can be run through this process. If operationalized, it can save the patient from unnecessary specimen collection and from medical bills for testing that will not be reimbursed.

Direct-to-provider Testing

In a typical send out process, a provider will order testing that is sent out through the Department of Pathology and Laboratory Medicine. The benefit of this system is that the laboratory has staff dedicated to this process that will ensure the specimen is sent to the appropriate laboratory in the right condition and that the results are entered in the patient's medical record. However, a form of testing that laboratories may not be aware of is that which is sent to the reference laboratory directly by the provider and circumvents the normal process for sending tests. Ideally, this testing would be regulated, monitored, and facilitated by the DSC but there are numerous challenges to be considered. First, capturing the full scope of this testing is difficult because Pathology and Laboratory Medicine is not handling the send out of the tests, thus, there is no data to be queried. In the absence of a report, DSCs can ask for providers to disclose what testing they are doing. This is far from a systematic evaluation and will certainly be incomplete. A second option is to go directly to the commercial laboratory performing the testing and ask that they provide a list of tests being done by your institution. This is also challenging because each individual provider will have set up agreements with the laboratories, and these agreements may or may not include the name of the institution making it difficult for the commercial laboratory to capture all the testing being done.

Another significant challenge with this testing is that because it does not go through official channels, in the laboratory, there is no mechanism for reliable result capture. Therefore, the results from these laboratories go directly back to the physician, often through a portal that is managed by the commercial laboratory. These portals help to expedite and simplify result reporting; however, they do pose potential risks of violating patient privacy. This is especially risky when the institution has not entered a formal contract with the commercial laboratory. In addition, these results do not have an official place to go in the patient's medical record, making it difficult for providers to locate and act up on the results.

Elements of billing and compliance can be difficult to understand with this kind of testing. Because there is no official contract with the institution and nonpathology departments do not typically pay for laboratory testing, commercial laboratories may be creative in how they obtain payment. Probably the most common is for the reference laboratory to manage payments. This is referred to as "third-party billing" and is a situation where the laboratory takes responsibility for billing, which means they will work with the patient's insurance or with the patient themselves to arrange payment. Another, perhaps more concerning scenario, is when the laboratory offers testing for free, typically in exchange for some form of enrollment in a research database. Free testing may also be offered on behalf of a pharmaceutical company because utilization of their drug is linked to the laboratory's test results. At face value, this may seem like a highly questionable practice but it has been reviewed by the Office of the Inspector general (OIG) and in advisory opinion No. 22-06 deemed acceptable (https://oig.hhs.gov/documents/advisory-opinions/1028/AO-22-06.pdf). In their discussion of the matter, the OIG states that in these circumstances, there is a clear separation between the pharmaceutical company and the testing laboratory and, therefore, does not violate the antikickback statutes.

Although there are clearly some concerning elements to this practice, the reality is these laboratories offer valuable testing that benefits patient care. These practices are firmly embedded in clinical practice and discontinuing them would have a negative impact on patient care. Unfortunately, although, the volume can be high and may be difficult for the laboratory to manage without adding staff. As a result, it may make sense for the laboratory to develop a hybrid send out model for these tests where providers may continue sending out the specimens directly but have orders built in the system. This would allow for some traceability and give the results a home in the medical record.

Regardless of the form direct-to-provider testing takes, it is something the DSC should be aware of and try to understand. We have found that these tests offer valuable options that our patients might not otherwise have. The DSC's goal should be to help facilitate this testing so that it can be done in a compliant manner and improve patient care by better capturing and presenting patient results.

Suggested Diagnostic Stewardship Interventions

Depending on the institution and the patient population, the DSC may have very different challenges to address. As a result, the following recommendations may not be suitable for all organizations but it is likely that some of the following ideas will present good opportunities for intervention and success; some have been discussed briefly earlier.

Multiplex polymerase chain reaction pathogen panels

Multiplex polymerase chain reaction (PCR) technology is now a commonplace in diagnostic laboratories. These tests, so-called syndromic panels, offer powerful capabilities to diagnose diseases for a wide variety of pathogens from a single specimen. They represent some of the most advanced diagnostic technology in the laboratory but come at a high cost. These panels allow providers to you order a single test with a high likelihood of getting a positive result. For example, it is not uncommon for more than 40% of respiratory pathogen panels to be positive.

There are a few reasons diagnostics stewardship committees may want to review these tests. First, they may be common sources of unnecessary repeat testing because they are ordered on patients presenting with respiratory symptoms and who are going to be admitted to the hospital. In reviewing our own data, we found a relatively high percentage of tests were repeated within a few hours of each other. On investigation, we learned that this was unintentional and that providers on the floors were ordering the test in duplicate because they were unaware that the emergency department had already ordered the test. Although it is probably appropriate to restrict repeat testing to several weeks, we were able to reduce a significant percentage of unnecessary repeat testing simply by setting a threshold of 24 hours, which virtually eliminated this problem.

In addition, recent local coverage determinants have outlined criteria for which this testing will not be reimbursed (https://www.cms.gov/medicare-coverage-database/view/lcd.aspx?lcdid=38916). Institutions will want to review their utilization to ensure the testing is being ordered in the right patient populations to avoid denial of payment. These are expensive reagents and high-volume tests that may cost the institution a significant amount of money if not being reimbursed.

Acetylcholine receptor cell-based assay

This test will be discussed as a representative example of testing which may pose challenges for DSCs. Acetylcholine receptor (AChR) cell-based assay detects antibodies in patients with myasthenia gravis with negative standard of care antibody results (radioimmunoprecipitation assay [RIPA]). For patients to be candidates for complement and neonatal crystallizable fragment receptor (FcRN) inhibitor treatments. It is estimated that ~20% of seronegative patients with myasthenia gravis will be positive by AChR testing.[7] This test is representative of a common challenge faced by committees with a variety of different competing interests. This test serves an important patient population but a relatively small one. It is offered by only a single laboratory in the United States but if positive connects these patients to desperately needed therapies that can treat their disease. The clinical utility of this testing is without question. However, the resources required to offer this are not trivial and come at the expense of other high-priority efforts. In addition, because the test is so new and only offered by a single laboratory, it is not currently reimbursable, so institutions supporting this testing will do so at a loss. This is an example of some of the difficult decisions the DSC must make. Newer committees may decide to table bringing on tests such as these until higher priorities have been accomplished.

Genomic diagnostics for infectious diseases

Culture negative results in patients with high suspicion for infectious diseases are a common occurrence and have led to the widespread adoption of culture independent diagnostics. The issue of culture-negativity is especially problematic in immunocompromised patients who are at high risk of bad outcomes. With an increasing number of vulnerable patients, there has been a sharp increase and utilization of genomic tests that can detect infectious diseases from various specimens. These diagnostics are powerful but also expensive and prone to misuse.

A relatively common situation encountered by laboratories is the surprise finding of a possible pathogen in histopathology when cultures have not been ordered. Without culture, clinicians can only guess as to what the infecting pathogen may be and what treatment would be best. In these circumstances, it may be appropriate to send the biopsy material for genomic analyses to determine the identity of the organism. In these situations, the specimen is sent to a laboratory, which will perform sequencing evaluation to try and identify the organism. These technologies have been around for a while and can yield impactful results. However, they are relatively low sensitivity and often fail to detect the pathogen. It is not appropriate to send this testing routinely, and it is especially low yield when the organism is not visualized by microscopy. DSCs could reasonably implement restrictions on this testing such that it will not be performed unless an organism is visualized, and culture results are negative.

More recently, the detection of cell-free DNA in circulating blood has grown in popularity.[8] In these tests, next generation sequencing methods detect cell-free DNA and identify pathogens. The concept is that as the host fights an infection, the pathogen's DNA is processed and circulates in the blood where it can be detected. This is a powerful technology but the diagnostic stewardship community is wrestling with how best to control its use. These tests can cost more than US$ 2000 and are usually ordered on inpatients and fall under the diagnosis-related group payment structure. At that price and at any moderate volume, these tests will quickly become the most expensive send out item for a laboratory. In addition, although some results are easy to interpret, a high percentage of tests yield complex and polymicrobial answers, which may lead to diagnostic confusion. There is a growing body of evidence looking at how best to use this test but the practical reality of it is that yearly expenditures can reach into the hundreds of thousands of dollars. It is recommended that DSCs establish an approval process for this testing, which engages key stakeholders such as infectious diseases and other groups such as bone marrow transplantation. Establishing strict criteria based on the literature will prove difficult but one strategy that may be effective is a "spin and hold" process where the testing can be ordered, and the

Table 1
Serologic tests prone to misuse

Serologic Testing	Diagnostic Stewardship Considerations
HSV IgM	Should never be done
Lyme disease, cerebrospinal fluid (CSF) Line Blot	Preferred diagnostic is IgG antibody index which compares antibody titers in the serum and CSF
H pylori	Not included in most diagnostic algorithms. High seropositivity make serology minimally useful
Bordetella pertussis IgM	Little diagnostic utility
Parvovirus B19 IgM and IgG	Should only rarely be used. IgM and IgG should not be ordered as standalone tests
Ehrlichia serology	PCR is the preferred diagnostic for acute disease. Serology should be rarely used
Brucella serology	Should only be ordered in patients with significant risk factors. Serology should be rarely used
Lyme serology	Prone to false-positive results. Should only be ordered in patients who are from or traveled to endemic areas

Abbreviations: HSV, herpes simplex virus; IgG, immunoglobulin G; IgM, immunoglobulin M.

specimen collected and held while routine cultures are given a chance to yield a result. If negative, then genomic cell-free testing can be sent. This is an advantageous workflow because it allows the providers to order and collect specimens at one moment in time and may reduce the risk of falsely negative results from specimens collected after antimicrobial therapy has been administered.

Serologic testing

A review of your laboratory's serologic testing may reveal surprising usage patterns. Especially in academic medical centers where unique diagnoses are considered by learners who are early in their training, serologic testing can often be misused. The following is a list of conditions for which serologic testing can be problematic and should be reviewed by the DSC (**Table 1**).

SUMMARY

This review summarizes various key elements of implementing an effective diagnostic stewardship program. The practice of diagnostic stewardship can take many forms and will need to be tailored to an institution's specific needs. Despite the tremendous variation in laboratory practices, this review discusses some common challenges that most institutions will encounter in their diagnostic stewardship efforts, such as how to identify wasteful/unnecessary testing practices and what to do about, how to handle prior authorization, reducing miscellaneous testing, direct-to-provider testing, and controlling reference laboratory testing.

DISCLOSURE

C.D. Doern – Shionogi, Quidel, Karius. C. Kidd: None.

REFERENCES

1. Beriault DR, Gilmour JA, Hicks LK. Overutilization in laboratory medicine: tackling the problem with quality improvement science. Crit Rev Clin Lab Sci 2021;58:430–46.

2. Doern CD. The confounding role of antimicrobial stewardship programs in understanding the impact of technology on patient care. J Clin Microbiol 2016;54: 2420–3.
3. Abbas S, Bernard S, Lee KB, et al. Rapid respiratory panel testing: impact of active antimicrobial stewardship. Am J Infect Control 2019;47:224–5.
4. MacMillan D, Lewandrowski E, Lewandrowski K. An analysis of reference laboratory (send out) testing: an 8-year experience in a large academic medical center. Clin Leader Manag Rev 2004;18:216–9.
5. Sanguinetti M, Posteraro B, Beigelman-Aubry C, et al. Diagnosis and treatment of invasive fungal infections: looking ahead. J Antimicrob Chemother 2019;74: ii27–37.
6. Smith HS, Franciskovich R, Lewis AM, et al. Outcomes of prior authorization requests for genetic testing in outpatient pediatric genetics clinics. Genet Med 2021;23:950–5.
7. Damato V, Spagni G, Monte G, et al. Clinical value of cell-based assays in the characterisation of seronegative myasthenia gravis. J Neurol Neurosurg Psychiatry 2022;93:995–1000.
8. Bell DT. Deciphering the potential of plasma cell-free metagenomic next-generation sequencing using the Karius test. Curr Opin Infect Dis 2023;36:420–5.

Home and Clinical Laboratory Improvement Amendments–Waived Testing for Infectious Diseases—How Do These Fit in the Testing Landscape?

Jacky Lu, PhD[a], Susan M. Butler-Wu, PhD[b,*]

KEYWORDS

• Clinical Laboratory Improvement Amendments • Antigen-based CLIA-waived testing
• Home or over-the-counter testing • Emergency use authorization

KEY POINTS

- The COVID-19 pandemic led to an unprecedented expansion in the availability of waived testing. This has led to renewed interest in this type of testing by both clinicians and the general public alike.
- The emergency use authorization pathway was also used for mpox medical countermeasures in the recent outbreak.
- Diagnostic stewardship and optimal test utilization of CLIA waived testing for infectious diseases is its infancy and is an area that requires greater development and resources.

It is clear that the coronavirus disease 2019 (COVID-19) pandemic has forever elevated the collective public consciousness and awareness of diagnostic testing for infectious diseases. The pandemic led to a boon of testing that can be performed outside of the traditional clinical laboratory environment. Though the pandemic has changed the public's perspective on what is possible in terms of diagnostic testing, testing for infectious diseases performed at home or in the clinic is not a new entity. Here, the authors discuss perspectives on the current landscape of clinical testing outside of the traditional laboratory environment and the role laboratory professionals can play in this setting.

[a] Department of Pathology and Laboratory Medicine, Children's Hospital Los Angeles, 4650 Sunset Boulevard, Los Angeles, CA 90027, USA; [b] Department of Pathology, Keck School of Medicine of the University of Southern California, HMR 211, 2011 Zonal Avenue, Los Angeles, CA 90033, USA
* Corresponding author.
E-mail address: SButler-Wu@dhs.lacounty.gov

Clin Lab Med 44 (2024) 13–21
https://doi.org/10.1016/j.cll.2023.10.005

CLINICAL LABORATORY IMPROVEMENT AMENDMENTS: NUTS AND BOLTS

The Clinical Laboratory Improvement Amendments of 1988 (CLIA) were implemented to ensure the accuracy and reliability of clinical laboratory testing in the United States.[1] These regulations were enacted in response to a wave of reports of inaccurate test results produced by diagnostic tools that were available at the time. This legislation impacts any setting that performs testing on human specimens for the purpose of diagnosis or treatment of an illness, disease, or assessment of the health of a person and includes, but is not limited to, hospitals, independent laboratories, and physician office laboratories. Non-laboratory patient care settings that perform clinical testing are considered laboratories under CLIA and generally must apply and obtain a certificate from the CLIA Program that corresponds to the complexity of the tests being performed (with the exception of laboratories in the states of New York and Washington).

Clinical testing that falls under CLIA regulation is separated into 3 categories based on test complexity: high-complexity, moderate-complexity, and waived testing. Following Food and Drug Administration (FDA) clearance or approval of a marketing submission or upon request for legally marketed devices, CLIA categorization is determined. The FDA determines the complexity of the test by reviewing the manufacturer's test instructions and uses a scorecard comprised of 7 criteria to determine testing complexity. These 7 criteria include (1) knowledge requirement of the operator, (2) training and experience, (3) reagents and materials, (4) characteristics of operational steps, (5) calibration, quality control, and proficiency testing materials, (6) test system troubleshooting and equipment maintenance, and (7) interpretation and judgment. Each of these criteria is scored between 1 and 3, from lowest to highest complexity. A total score of less than 12 is considered moderate complexity, while scores over 12 are designated as high complexity.

Waived tests are defined by CLIA as "*simple laboratory examinations and procedures that have an insignificant risk of an erroneous result*" as determined by the Code of Federal Regulations [ie, 42 CFR 493.15(c)]. The test must be approved by the FDA, employ methodologies that are simple and accurate enough to almost eliminate inaccurate results, and be one for which the Secretary of Health and Human Services has determined that incorrectly performed tests pose no reasonable risk to the patient.[2] The FDA determines which tests meet these criteria when it reviews a manufacturer's application for a test system waiver and these waived tests bypass the complexity score described earlier.[3]

Home or over-the-counter (OTC) testing refers to self-administered tests that are cleared by the FDA for home use and, as a result, do not generally fall under CLIA regulations. This class of testing refers to tests where both specimen collection and testing are performed by a single individual. In contrast, home-collected specimens are self-collected by an individual but require testing (ie, processing and analysis) by another party such as a reference laboratory. If a test is classified as OTC but another individual is doing either the testing or interpretation of the results, then a CLIA certificate would be required. The global COVID-19 pandemic resulted in the widespread use of an alternative regulatory pathway at the FDA for tests of all complexity levels for severe acute respiratory syndrome coronavirus 2 (SARS-CoV-2) detection, including home use: emergency use authorization (EUA). This allowed the FDA to authorize the use of unapproved medical countermeasures (MCMs), in anticipation of a potential emergency or during an actual emergency involving a chemical, biological, radiological, or nuclear agent, or an emerging infectious disease.[4] The EUA pathway was also used for mpox MCMs in the recent outbreak.

CURRENT LANDSCAPE OF CLINICAL LABORATORY IMPROVEMENT AMENDMENTS–WAIVED TESTING FOR INFECTIOUS DISEASES TESTING

What Is Old Is New Again: Antigen-Based Clinical Laboratory Improvement Amendments–Waived Testing

There are hundreds of tests with CLIA-waived status for a variety of indications, including several that look for signs of infection (eg, urine dipstick, fecal occult blood) according to the FDA's publicly available database. Of these, there are over 250 for infectious diseases at the time of writing. CLIA-waived tests that look for antibody response include human immunodeficiency virus (HIV), hepatitis C, syphilis, and Lyme disease. There are also over 60 CLIA-waived tests with EUA that test for SARS-CoV-2 either alone or in combination with other respiratory pathogens.[5]

The use of CLIA-waived testing for antibody detection has been available for many years (eg, for HIV). In general, results from CLIA-waived serologic tests are considered preliminary in nature and require confirmation with laboratory-based tests such as enzyme immunoassays, Western blots, or even polymerase chain reactions (PCRs). Point-of-care testing for HIV, though less sensitive compared to traditional testing, is associated with increased rates of testing for HIV and delivery of HIV status results to patients, compared to conventional laboratory-based HIV testing.[5]

Detection of pathogen antigens has been a mainstay of CLIA-waived testing for many years. Though this is relatively more affordable than other testing modalities and often does not require specialized equipment, antigen tests are generally less sensitive than culture or nucleic acid amplification testing (NAAT). Though this position has generated some degree of controversy over the course of the COVID-19 pandemic, this phenomenon has been well described for many years for a range of antigen-based tests and pathogens. It is neither surprising nor a newly observed phenomenon that antigen tests have generally lower sensitivities than NAAT. For instance, though the College of American Pathologists only requires backup throat culture in children testing negative for group A *Streptococcus* (GAS) by rapid antigen testing, package inserts for several of these assays require that backup throat culture be performed. The use of rapid GAS antigen testing as a stand-alone diagnostic is therefore considered an off-label use of these tests and requires validation. Studies have repeatedly shown poorer sensitivity for antigen-based GAS tests compared to culture.[6] In contrast, the performance of CLIA-waived antigen-based testing for *Helicobacter pylori* performed on stool (ImmunoCard STAT HpSA) showed a sensitivity and specificity of 92.6% and 88.5%, respectively, with an overall accuracy of 90.6%.[7]

Beyond bacteria, similar findings of suboptimal test performance have also been described for several viral infections most notably during the emergence of novel H1N1 influenza A. Several meta-analyses have been published regarding the performance of CLIA-waived antigen testing for influenza viruses and showed pooled sensitivities of 64.6% and 52.5% for influenza A and B, respectively, with pooled specificities of 98.2%.[8] Though the use of digital readers has improved performance, sensitivities are still in the order of 80%. Consequently, the US Centers for Disease Control (CDC) has continued to recommend that confirmatory testing of negative specimens be performed when influenza infection is clinically suspected. A similar phenomenon has also been noted for antigen testing for SARS-CoV-2. A meta-analysis of 152 studies looking at 228 evaluations of rapid antigen tests for SARS-CoV-2 showed sensitivities of 73% among symptomatic individuals.[9] A subsequent study found that package inserts for rapid antigen tests overestimated sensitivities compared to real-world analyses.[10]

Fundamentally, the sensitivity of antigen-based testing is determined by the amount of pathogen antigen that is present in the sample, and antigen tests have almost universally higher limits of detection than methods that rely on nucleic acid detection. Consequently, for respiratory viruses, antigen tests are more likely to be positive in specimens with higher viral loads. However, this phenomenon crosses microbial kingdoms and is also observed for malarial and bacterial antigen detection.[11] Ultimately, the FDA only requires demonstration of sensitivity greater than 80% for SARS-CoV-2 antigen tests and allows for sensitivities even lower than this when a serial testing strategy is used.[12]

New School: the Emergence of Clinical Laboratory Improvement Amendments–Waived Molecular Testing

There has been an increase in the number of CLIA-waived NAATs in recent years. In addition to improved analytical and clinical sensitivities, these also consequently have higher negative predictive values compared to antigen-based tests. The performance of CLIA-waived PCRs is generally equivalent to laboratory-based testing. For instance, results of the cobas Liat Strep A assay (Roche Diagnostics, Indianapolis, IN, USA) showed an overall concordance of 97.2% with laboratory-based PCR testing among 468 subjects tested in duplicate.[13] Nevertheless, just as with antigen-based tests, not all NAATs perform identically. An illustration of this was shown by Kanwar and colleagues who compared the performance of 3 CLIA-waived influenza NAATs: ID NOW Influenza A & B 2 (Abbott, IL, USA; formerly known as Alere i influenza A/B 2), cobas Influenza A/B (Liat; Roche Molecular Systems, Inc., Indianapolis, IN, USA), and Xpert Xpress Flu (Cepheid, Sunnydale, CA, USA). The performance of these 3 assays was compared with the BD Veritor Flu A/B antigen test (BD Diagnostics, Sparks, MD, USA) in children with the CDC Flu A/B PCR serving as the reference method.[14] From a cohort of 201 children between the ages of 0 and 200 months (median age of 42 months) with suspected upper respiratory infections, the sensitivities for influenza A and B detection, respectively, were as follows: 93.2%/97.2% for the ID NOW assay, 100%/94.4% for the Liat assay, and 100%/91.7% for the Xpert assay. In contrast, the sensitivity of the BD antigen assay was 79.5%/66.7%. The specificities for influenza A and B virus detection were greater than 97% for all assays.

One area for greater deployment of CLIA-waived molecular testing is in the diagnosis of sexually transmitted infections (STIs) where the incidence of these infections has been increasing year-over-year in the United States for the last 5 years.[15,16] The first CLIA-waived assays for *Chlamydia* and gonorrhea were approved in the United States in 2021. The availability of such assays has the potential to improve detection and treatment rates for STIs in the United States. In a study from England where *Chlamydia* and gonorrhea point-of-care testing was used in 3 clinics, reduced time to treatment and a reduction in unnecessary treatment for *Chlamydia* were observed.[17] The recent availability of CLIA-waived molecular assays that include *Trichomonas vaginalis* is an important development in this space for female patients as *T vaginalis* is known to be underdiagnosed using non–molecular-based methods.[18] Future potential inclusion of *T vaginalis* in approved assays for male patients has the potential to further prevent partner transmission as part of routine sexual health testing. In October 2023, Cepheid Xpert Xpress MVP received CLIA-waived status for an assay that detects bacterial vaginosis (BV), vulvovaginal candidiasis, and trichomoniasis. However, the high rate of detection of BV organisms in completely asymptomatic black and Latino women raises concerns over the possibility of overtreatment and overdiagnosis of this infection, particularly in non–clinic-based CLIA-waived settings, for example, pharmacies and mobile testing laboratories.

One of the advantages of CLIA-waived rapid molecular testing is its relative ease of use. In contrast, high-complexity molecular testing requires highly trained licensed staff, equipment, and resources that are limited to microbiology or reference laboratories. The increasing availability of CLIA-waived PCR tests has the potential to further democratize access to high-sensitivity molecular testing. Such tests can now be performed outside of the clinical laboratory with appropriately trained non-laboratory operators, such as in physicians' offices, urgent care centers, outreach clinics, pharmacies, as well as in temporary patient care settings such as mobile laboratories. Nevertheless, concerns have been raised regarding the deployment of highly sensitive methods such as PCR in the hands of personnel who are not specially trained in molecular techniques. Though not well studied, Shihabuddin and colleagues evaluated the performance of the Cepheid Xpert Xpress Flu/RSV (Cepheid, Sunnydale, CA, USA) in a CLIA-waived setting with minimally trained non-laboratory operators.[19] Testing personnel were non-laboratory health care staff with no prior experience using the GeneXpert or any other moderately complex test platform. All personnel (n = 44) were provided only with the reference guides included with the commercial kits and test system and were not specifically trained on the operation of either the GeneXpert Xpress System or the Xpert Xpress Flu/RSV test. The ease of use of the test was evaluated by a 23-question survey. With a score of 1 representing strongly disagree to 5 representing strongly agree, the average scores for all questions regarding ease of use and understanding of the results were above 4 indicate that CLIA-waived testing and likely other similar types of assays are user friendly.

Another potential concern with the use of highly sensitive CLIA-waived molecular tests is the potential for contamination leading to false-positive results. Though CLIA-waived NAATs are generally "closed systems," there is reasonable concern that the surrounding environment could potentially become contaminated by the specimens being tested at the point of device inoculation. Though this has not been extensively studied, the risk of environmental contamination leading to false-positive results was addressed in one study looking at the performance of the CLIA-waived Cobas Liat Strep A assay. From 26 swabs collected around the instrument over the course of testing on 400 patients, no environmental contamination with GAS deoxyribonucleic acid was detected suggesting minimal contamination risk with use of this assay.[13]

As the technology has evolved, many CLIA-waived molecular tests have extremely rapid turnaround times, approaching or, in some cases, being lower than those of antigen-based tests. Consequently, results are dramatically faster than when testing is performed in off-site laboratories where specimens must first be transported to the testing location, which is a common practice for many doctors' offices and clinics. Examples of this include the ID NOW platform where some assays have a 5-minute turnaround time,[14] the cobas Liat analyzer which provides results within 20 minutes, and the GeneXpert system which markets a 30-minute turnaround time. The increasing availability of decentralized CLIA-waived rapid molecular tests facilitates testing that is close to the patient, thus improving treatment decision-making and in turn having the potential to reduce onward transmission. Influenza guidelines recommend initiation of antivirals within 48 hours of symptom onset for optimal response.[20] Similarly, antivirals for COVID-19 (eg, nirmatrelvir and ritonavir [Paxlovid]) must also be initiated within 5 days of symptoms.[21] Because patients infrequently present for care upon initial symptoms, the window of opportunity in which to begin treatment is automatically shortened. It is in such settings that CLIA-waived testing can make a real difference, extending the effective treatment window compared to traditional laboratory-based testing.

Rapid diagnosis by molecular testing in hospital-based settings has been shown to reduce the length of hospitalization as well as the duration of unnecessary antibiotics and unnecessary imaging.[22] The impact of CLIA-waived testing in clinic settings has begun to be investigated. In a single-center study performed at the NorthShore University HealthSystem, CLIA-waived testing led to a reduction in inappropriate antiviral prescriptions by 10.8% (2.3% vs 13.1%) compared to the standard CLIA-waived algorithm comprised of antigen testing with reflex for PCR testing for negative results (associated with turnaround time of an additional 48 hours).[23] The longer turnaround time associated with confirmatory PCR in this setting also required additional logistic and financial costs which were eliminated with CLIA-waived testing. These data show that the use of CLIA-waived assays can positively contribute to improved antimicrobial stewardship.

From the perspective of patients, ready accessibility to CLIA-waived testing can be extremely beneficial by bringing testing closer to the patient. Traditional health care settings such as hospitals and clinics can be out of the way for some communities with access to transportation challenging for many patients. Travel to health care settings can also be emotionally taxing, resulting in decreased productivity and even wages. This can also require planning for childcare and potentially even increase the likelihood of transmitting the pathogen to other individuals in the process of transportation, for example, public transport. Rapid access to decentralized testing can, therefore, also reduce the cost of unnecessary prescriptions by reducing the use of unnecessary empiric therapy, which can be a burden especially to communities and populations without insurance.

HOME-BASED INFECTIOUS DISEASE TESTING

Prior to the pandemic, home-based testing for infectious diseases (ie, testing performed and resulted within the home) was limited in the United States to HIV antibody detection. Now, the US market has a relatively large number of commercially available home-based tests for SARS-CoV-2, both antigen and molecular. Though the availability of home-based testing in theory offers a fully democratized process, facilitating an "anytime anywhere" approach, the sensitivity of testing performed in the home is lower than that performed in health care settings. In one study, the sensitivity of rapid antigen testing for SARS-CoV-2 performed by self-trained members of the public was 57.5% compared with 70% for fully trained research health care workers.[23] In contrast, the highest sensitivity in this study was observed for laboratory scientists (78.8%). Though antigen testing is a somewhat less forgiving method in terms of the relationship between degree of test positivity and the amount of antigen present in the sample, the same trend was also observed for collection of specimens for molecular testing. In one study looking at home-collected samples that were testing in a clinical laboratory, the sensitivity was only 80% compared with specimens collected by clinicians. These data suggest that testing collected and performed in the home, including molecular testing, is likely to be somewhat reduced in sensitivity compared to testing performed in a CLIA-waived or a laboratory environment.

The aforementioned impact on test sensitivity has ramifications for undertreatment and onward spread of infectious diseases. The CDC currently recommends that at-home COVID-19 antigen testing be repeated after 48 hours in patients with COVID-19 symptoms (ie, serial testing). Studies have begun to show that the general public does not always fully understand the significance of negative results[24] and that the public perception of testing can change over time.[25] A further concern, which has been realized with the increasing availability of at-home COVID-19 testing, is underreporting of positive results to public health authorities.[26] Though home testing for STIs beyond HIV has not yet been realized in the United States, underreporting and lack of linkage to care is a potential concern in this space.

THE ONLY THING CONSTANT IS CHANGE: THE EVOLUTION OF THE ROLE OF THE MEDICAL MICROBIOLOGIST AND OTHER LABORATORY SPECIALISTS IN THIS CHANGING LANDSCAPE

The rise of CLIA-waived testing for infectious diseases might have many wondering if this is the death knell of traditional laboratory testing. Ultimately, as long as hospitals exist, so too will testing performed in clinical laboratories. Clinical laboratories increasingly use the moderate-complexity version of CLIA-waived tests to harness the impact of rapid test turnaround times. Although specimen transport increases time to results overall, many hospitals possess the infrastructure to rapidly deliver specimens to the diagnostic clinical laboratories, including microbiology. Decentralization of some tests throughout a health care enterprise by deployment of CLIA-waived testing can reduce the pressure on clinical laboratories which continue to face an interminable shortage of licensed clinical laboratory scientists.

However, the increasing penetrance of CLIA-waived testing in health care systems should not reduce the involvement of laboratory personnel in the process but rather change the nature of this involvement. Deployment of CLIA-waived testing, particularly molecular-based testing, across health care systems requires immense financial investment. As a result, the price of performing these assays may be higher compared to more conventional laboratory-based testing which must be offset through improved patient outcomes and reductions in the use of resources. It is here that the involvement and oversight of laboratory professionals should be paramount. The resources required to ensure compliance with CLIA-waived regulations are not trivial. The knowledge and experience to run such programs are not typically taught to other medical professions. In contrast, these come naturally and are part and parcel of the practice of clinical laboratory professionals.

It is the authors' position that laboratory professionals, including medical microbiologists, should be responsible for oversight of CLIA-waived testing for infectious diseases including the oversight of quality. This also includes diagnostic test stewardship and working with clinical colleagues to mitigate against off-label use of these devices. Nowhere is this more paramount than in the case of syndromic testing for infections which is likely to increasingly have CLIA-waived tests available.

It is evident that CLIA-waived testing, particularly molecular-based testing, is here to stay and will increasingly become the new normal as adoption of these technologies spread. This development has the potential to increase equity of care by making diagnostic testing more readily available, ideally when tied to linkage to care. However, without the involvement of laboratory professionals in this process, appropriate monitoring and assurance of quality will be challenging to ensure. It is therefore only with the continued involvement of laboratory professionals in the form of appropriate management and oversight that patients will be able to rely on the same quality of testing they have come to expect from traditional laboratory-based testing.

REFERENCES

1. Centers for Medicare & Medicaid Services. CLIA Regulations and Federal Register Documents. Available at: https://www.cms.gov/medicare/quality/clinical-laboratory-improvement-amendments/regulations-federal-register. Accessed October 9, 2023.
2. Babady NE, Dunn JJ, Madej R. CLIA-waived molecular influenza testing in the emergency department and outpatient settings. J Clin Virol 2019;116. https://doi.org/10.1016/j.jcv.2019.05.002.

3. Zhang JY, Bender AT, Boyle DS, et al. Current state of commercial point-of-care nucleic acid tests for infectious diseases. Analyst 2021;146(8). https://doi.org/10.1039/d0an01988g.
4. Mitchell SL, St George K, Rhoads DD, et al. Understanding, verifying, and implementing emergency use authorization molecular diagnostics for the detection of sars-cov-2 RNA. J Clin Microbiol 2020;58(8). https://doi.org/10.1128/JCM.00796-20.
5. Pottie K, Medu O, Welch V, et al. Effect of rapid HIV testing on HIV incidence and services in populations at high risk for HIV exposure: an equity-focused systematic review. BMJ Open 2014;4(12). https://doi.org/10.1136/bmjopen-2014-006859.
6. Kim HN, Kim J, Jang WS, et al. Performance evaluation of three rapid antigen tests for the diagnosis of group A Streptococci. BMJ Open 2019;9(8). https://doi.org/10.1136/bmjopen-2018-025438.
7. Hsu J, Santesso N, Mustafa R, et al. Antivirals for treatment of influenza: a systematic review and meta-analysis of observational studies. Ann Intern Med 2012; 156(7). https://doi.org/10.7326/0003-4819-156-7-201204030-00411.
8. Chartrand C, Leeflang MMG, Minion J, et al. Accuracy of rapid influenza diagnostic tests: a meta-analysis. Ann Intern Med 2012;156(7). https://doi.org/10.7326/0003-4819-156-7-201204030-00403.
9. Dinnes J, Sharma P, Berhane S, et al. Rapid, point-of-care antigen tests for diagnosis of SARS-CoV-2 infection. Cochrane Database Syst Rev 2022;(7):2022. https://doi.org/10.1002/14651858.CD013705.pub3.
10. Bigio J, MacLean ELH, Das R, et al. Accuracy of package inserts of SARS-CoV-2 rapid antigen tests: a secondary analysis of manufacturer versus systematic review data. Lancet Microbe 2023. https://doi.org/10.1016/S2666-5247(23)00222-7.
11. Yimam Y, Mohebali M, Abbaszadeh Afshar MJ. Comparison of diagnostic performance between conventional and ultrasensitive rapid diagnostic tests for diagnosis of malaria: a systematic review and meta-analysis. PLoS One 2022;17(2): e0263770.
12. Food and Drug Administration. Template for Developers of Antigen Tests. 2021.
13. Donato LJ, Myhre NK, Murray MA, et al. Assessment of test performance and potential for environmental contamination associated with a point-of-care molecular assay for group A Streptococcus in an end user setting. J Clin Microbiol 2019; 57(2). https://doi.org/10.1128/JCM.01629-18.
14. Kanwar N, Michael J, Doran K, et al. Comparison of the ID now influenza A & B 2, cobas influenza A/B, and xpert xpress flu point-of-care nucleic acid amplification tests for influenza A/B virus detection in children. J Clin Microbiol 2020;58(3). https://doi.org/10.1128/JCM.01611-19.
15. CDC. Sexually Transmitted Diseases (STDs): Date and Statistics. Published April 11, 2023. Accessed October 20, 2023. https://www.cdc.gov/std/statistics/default.htm.
16. Huntington S, Weston G, Adams E. Assessing the clinical impact and resource use of a 30-minute chlamydia and gonorrhoea point-of-care test at three sexual health services. Ther Adv Infect Dis 2021;8. https://doi.org/10.1177/20499361211061645.
17. Roth AM, Williams JA, Ly R, et al. Changing sexually transmitted infection screening protocol will result in improved case finding for trichomonas vaginalis among high-risk female populations. Sex Transm Dis 2011;38(5):398–400.

18. Shihabuddin BS, Faron ML, Relich RF, et al. Cepheid Xpert Xpress Flu/RSV evaluation performed by minimally trained non-laboratory operators in a CLIA-waived environment. Diagn Microbiol Infect Dis 2022;104(2).
19. Andrews D, Chetty Y, Cooper BS, et al. Multiplex PCR point of care testing versus routine, laboratory-based testing in the treatment of adults with respiratory tract infections: a quasi-randomised study assessing impact on length of stay and antimicrobial use. BMC Infect Dis 2017;17(1). https://doi.org/10.1186/s12879-017-2784-z.
20. Garg N, Kunamneni AS, Garg P, et al. Antiviral drugs and vaccines for omicron variant: a focused review. Can J Infect Dis Med Microbiol 2023. https://doi.org/10.1155/2023/6695533.
21. Rappo U, Schuetz AN, Jenkins SG, et al. Impact of early detection of respiratory viruses by multiplex PCR assay on clinical outcomes in adult patients. J Clin Microbiol 2016;54(8). https://doi.org/10.1128/JCM.00549-16.
22. Peto T, Affron D, Afrough B, et al. COVID-19: rapid antigen detection for SARS-CoV-2 by lateral flow assay: a national systematic evaluation of sensitivity and specificity for mass-testing. EClinicalMedicine 2021;36. https://doi.org/10.1016/j.eclinm.2021.100924.
23. McCulloch DJ, Kim AE, Wilcox NC, et al. Comparison of unsupervised home self-collected midnasal swabs with clinician-collected nasopharyngeal swabs for detection of SARS-CoV-2 infection. JAMA Netw Open 2020;3(7):e2016382.
24. Woloshin S, Dewitt B, Krishnamurti T, et al. Assessing how consumers interpret and act on results from at-home COVID-19 self-test kits: a randomized clinical trial. JAMA Intern Med 2022;182(3):332–41.
25. Gavurova B, Ivankova V, Rigelsky M, et al. Perception of COVID-19 testing in the entire population. Front Public Health 2022;10:757065.
26. Park S, Marcus GM, Olgin JE, et al. Unreported SARS-CoV-2 home testing and test positivity. JAMA Netw Open 2023;6(1):e2252684.

Point of Care Molecular Testing

Current State and Opportunities for Diagnostic Stewardship

Caitlin Otto, PhD[a,*], Dan Chen, PhD[a]

KEYWORDS

• Point of care • Molecular test • Diagnostic stewardship

KEY POINTS

- Many molecular tests are now FDA-cleared for use in a point-of-care (POC) setting, offering highly sensitive tests for use at the patient bedside.
- Implementation of molecular tests in POC settings has created new challenges for ensuring the tests are used appropriately.
- There are opportunities and challenges for establishing diagnostic stewardship programs for molecular testing performed in the POC setting.

INTRODUCTION

In an effort to control hospital-acquired infections, the United States Centers for Medicare and Medicaid services (CMS) mandated that by 2017 all hospitals implement an antimicrobial stewardship program (ASP) to promote the optimization of antibiotic use. Since that time, diagnostic stewardship programs have also been implemented at many hospitals to work synergistically with ASP programs as an upstream effort to provide the right test, for the right patient, at the right time.[1,2]

Diagnostic stewardship is the set of coordinated guidance and interventions used to help direct the appropriate utilization of laboratory testing to ultimately guide patient management and treatment decisions.[3,4] Diagnostic stewardship programs involve pre-analytical, analytical, and post-analytical processes to modify the process of ordering, collecting, performing, and reporting of diagnostic tests with the overall goal to optimize clinical outcomes and limit the spread of antimicrobial resistance.[5] An important distinction is that the goal of diagnostic stewardship is not to simply limit

[a] Department of Pathology, New York University Langone Health, 560 1st Avenue, New York, NY 10016, USA
* Corresponding author.
E-mail address: Caitlin.Otto@nyulangone.org

Clin Lab Med 44 (2024) 23–32
https://doi.org/10.1016/j.cll.2023.10.010

the total number of tests that are completed, but rather to optimize the use of the *right test* in the *right clinical scenario*.

Inappropriate ordering practices by either under or over ordering diagnostic testing are recognized problems that can have negative downstream consequences.[6] The interpretation of a test result depends on the pre-test probability of disease; the post-test probability of disease increases as the pre-test probability increases. Likewise, the post-test probability decreases as the pre-test probability decreases. The interpretation of a test result cannot be done without considering the known patient factors prior to performing the test. The influence of pre-test probability on a test result is magnified by the increased use of sensitive molecular tests and molecular syndromic panels. The over reliance on these highly sensitive and specific tests can ultimately lead to inaccurate results, excessive antimicrobial exposure, and potentially other negative downstream consequences, such as adverse drug events, *Clostridioides difficile* infection, and selective pressure leading to development of resistance.[4,7]

While conventional clinical microbiology diagnostics are relatively inexpensive, molecular tests are more costly. The price of molecular-based tests has been increasing by 15% to 20% relative to an average of 4% to 5% for all health care costs, further elevating the need to address their clinical value.[8] While the goal of new clinical tests is to improve patient outcomes, their broad use alone cannot accomplish this goal. Misuse of these tests can add unnecessary costs and can ultimately lead to incorrect diagnoses and inappropriate treatment.[5]

The Food and Drug Administration (FDA) classifies testing into waived and non-waived tests. Waived tests are defined by Clinical Laboratory Improvement Amendments (CLIA) as those that are simple to perform with a low risk for an incorrect result.[9] Nonwaived tests are further subdivided into moderate and high complexity and must be performed in a CLIA-approved laboratory by licensed personnel. Laboratories performing non-waived tests are subjected to stringent CLIA regulations and are regularly inspected. Molecular-based infectious diseases testing has historically been classified as high complexity and was exclusively performed in high-complexity laboratory setting. However, the first infectious disease CLIA-waived molecular point of care test (POCT) was FDA-cleared in 2015, opening the door for molecular testing to be performed at the patient bedside. Since that time, molecular POCT utilization has increased, necessitating a thoughtful review of their utility and appropriate utilization in these new settings.

Implementation of diagnostic stewardship programs has helped to address the testing strategies in hospital-based settings; however, they have largely been absent in the point-of-care (POC) setting. Now due to the availability of high-cost molecular testing in the POC setting, the appropriate utilization of these tests has increasingly become a focus of attention. Molecular testing in the POC setting presents unique challenges for diagnostic stewardship initiatives. In this article, we will discuss the available molecular POC tests and opportunities and challenges for establishing diagnostic stewardship programs for molecular testing performed in the POC setting.

MOLECULAR POINT-OF-CARE TESTS

Point-of-care testing is testing that is performed near the site of patient care. The testing is often performed by licensed, non-laboratory health care personnel at a location outside of laboratory, but may also be performed by laboratory personnel.[10] Testing may be performed near the patient bedside within a hospital, in nursing homes, or in any other outpatient settings (eg, physician offices).[11] POCT may involve the use of either CLIA-waived or moderate complexity categories tests, which is determined by the FDA based on the complexity of the test, stability of calibrators, controls, and preanalytical steps.

Point-of-care testing for infectious diseases such as influenza, respiratory syncytial virus (RSV), or group-A *Streptococcus* (GAS) has historically consisted of CLIA-waived, rapid antigen tests.[12–14] Antigen tests have the advantage of a short turn-around time (TAT), they are easy to perform, and typically do not require special equipment to use. POC molecular tests are likewise easy to use, have a short turn-around time, but do require an instrument. The sensitivity of antigen tests is generally low, relative to their molecular counterparts. Comparisons of waived molecular tests to antigen consistently demonstrate marked improvement in sensitivity of molecular tests over antigen tests. In 1 such example, the Quidel QuckVue in line strep A antigen test only detected 5.2% of culture-positive specimens, relative to a 95.2% to 100% sensitivity of a panel of waived molecular tests for GAS.[15] It is largely due to this increase in sensitivity and specificity that has driven the rapid expansion of molecular testing in POC settings.

The introduction of molecular diagnostics in the POC setting has changed the paradigms for diagnosis and treatment of infections. The Infectious Diseases Society of America (IDSA) now recommends molecular assays over antigen tests for influenza testing in outpatients. Treatment of influenza in hospitalized patients is recommended without waiting for the result of any diagnostic testing, regardless of methodology. However, when testing for influenza in inpatients, IDSA recommends using molecular test. Rapid diagnosis of viral infections can expedite discontinuation of unnecessary antibiotics, inform antiviral use for respiratory virus infections, and in a hospital-based setting can help guide infection control decisions.[16]

The first test based on nucleic acid amplification to be granted a CLIA waiver was the Alere i influenza A & B test, which was approved in January 2015. This assay employs a nicking endonuclease amplification reaction, isothermal amplification with influenza-specific primers, followed by target detection with molecular beacon probes. This assay differentiates influenza A from B, requires 2 min to set up and process 1 nasal swab sample, and requires a total of 15 min to complete.[17,18] The assay sensitivity and specificity compared with that of viral cell culture in a seven-site clinical study were 97.8% and 85.6%, respectively, for influenza type A and 91.8% and 96.3%, respectively, for influenza type B.[17,19] Since approval of the Alere i influena A & B test, many other tests have been CLIA waived through the FDA (**Table 1**).

The BioFire FilmArray Respiratory Panel EZ 2.0 received CLIA waived status by the FDA in 2016 as the first and only CLIA-waived syndromic molecular panel that detects both bacterial and viral respiratory targets. The FilmArray respiratory panel EZ 2.0 detects the following 15 viral and 4 bacterial respiratory pathogens simultaneously from nasopharyngeal swabs: adenovirus, coronavirus 229E, coronavirus HKU1, coronavirus NL63, coronavirus OC43, severe acute respiratory syndrome coronavirus 2 (SARS-CoV-2), human metapneumovirus (MPV), human rhinovirus/enterovirus, influenza A, influenza A subtype H1, influenza A subtype H3, influenza A subtype H1-2009, influenza B, parainfluenza virus, respiratory syncytial virus, *Bordetella pertussis*, *Bordetella parapertussis*, *Chlamydophila pneumoniae*, and *Mycoplasma pneumoniae*. The FilmArray is a closed system that performs automated nucleic acid extraction, reverse transcription, nucleic acid amplification from a single nasopharyngeal specimen, and results analysis in approximately 45 minutes per specimen. A minimum of 300 μL nasopharyngeal specimen collected into viral transport media is needed for each run. The user places the specimen into the pouch and loads it into the instrument where all other operations are automated.[20]

Table 1
Summary of clinical laboratory improvement amendments-waived molecular tests for infectious diseases[22]

Manufacturer	Instrument	Test Name	Targets	Sample Types
Respiratory Infections				
Abbott	ID NOW	ID NOW RSV	Viral	Nasal swab
		ID NOW Influenza A & B 2	Viral	Nasal swab Nasopharyngeal swab
		ID NOW STREP A 2	Bacterial	Throat swab
		ID NOW COVID-19 2.0	Viral	Nasal swab Nasopharyngeal swab
Biofire Diagnostics	FilmArray 2.0	FilmArray Respiratory Panel 2.0 EZ	Bacterial Viral	Nasopharyngeal swab
	SPOTFIRE	Respiratory panel mini	Bacterial Viral	Nasopharyngeal swab
Cepheid	GeneXpert	Xpert Xpress Strep A	Bacterial	Throat swab
		Xpert Xpress CoV-2 plus	Viral	Nasal swab Nasopharyngeal swab
		Xpert Xpress CoV-2 plus	Viral	Nasal swab Nasopharyngeal swab
		Xpert Xpress Flu	Viral	Nasal swab Nasopharyngeal swab
Cue Health Inc	Cue Reader	Cue COVID-19 Molecular test	Viral	Nasal swab
ThermoFisher	Accula Dock	Accula SARS-CoV-2 Test	Viral	Nasal swab
		Accula Flu A/Flu B	Viral	Nasal swab
Roche Molecular	cobas LIAT	cobas SARS-CoV-2	Viral	Nasal swab Nasopharyngeal swab Mid-turbinate swab
		cobas SARS-CoV-2 & Influenza A/B	Viral	Nasal swab Nasopharyngeal swab
		cobas Strep A	Bacterial	Throat swab
Sexually-transmitted infections				
Binx Health	binx io	*Neisseria gonorrhoeae* *Chlamydia*	Bacterial	Vaginal swab Urine, male
Visby Medical, Inc	Visby medical Sexual Health	*Neisseria gonorrhoeae* *Chlamydia* *Trichomonas*	Bacterial Parasitic	Self-collected vaginal swabs

From Administration UFD. Devices@FDA. Accessed 10/26/2023, https://www.accessdata.fda.gov/scripts/cdrh/devicesatfda/index.cfm.

The newest category of molecular testing in the POC space is targeting sexually transmitted infections. In 2021, Binx Health was the first company to receive approval for a CLIA-waived test that detects *Neisseria gonorrhoeae* and *Chlamydia* in self-collected vaginal swabs and male urine. A 2020 trial demonstrated a sensitivity for

Chlamydia of 96.1% for women and 92.5% for men. For gonorrhea, the sensitivity estimates were 100.0% for women and 97.3% for men. This study also compared the performance of self-collected to provider-collected vaginal swabs and demonstrated an equivalent performance between the 2 collection strategies.[21] STI testing in the POC setting has the potential to decrease community prevalence by reducing the time to treatment and expediting partner notification. However, POC testing may create a gap in communicable disease surveillance data given the current dependence on mandated data reporting from clinical laboratories.

Overall, the availability and utilization of POC molecular tests has greatly increased since their introduction in 2015. Currently, there are 17 CLIA-waived molecular tests on the market for infectious diseases, summarized in **Table 1**, and others in development.

ADVANTAGES OF PERFORMING MOLECULAR TESTING IN A POINT-OF-CARE SETTING

Turn-Around Time to Results

Molecular microbiology has revolutionized clinical infectious disease diagnostics. The TAT for laboratory-based respiratory virus testing has decreased from days with viral culture to hours with the use of molecular tests. Point-of-care respiratory testing was previously available with a TAT of 15 to 20 minutes; however, the low sensitivity of antigen tests limited their clinical utility. Now, the availability of POC molecular testing for respiratory viruses has reduced the TAT of high-quality respiratory virus testing, to as few as 15 minutes in some cases. Likewise, the length of time for Group A *Streptococcus* diagnosis can take 1 to 2 days. Due to the low sensitivity of antigen tests, POC group A *Streptococcus* screening requires a reflex culture if the antigen test is negative.[23] A distinct advantage of molecular testing for GAS is that a reflex culture is not required. Molecular testing can be performed in a high-complexity laboratory or at POC; however, as with the respiratory virus testing, the total TAT to results is faster if done at the POC. Molecular POC for GAS enables clinicians to diagnose and treat patients during the same visit.[24] Rao and colleagues determined that the use of molecular POCTs resulted in the appropriate prescribing of antibiotics in 97.1% of cases, compared to 87.5% of cases utilizing rapid antigen testing followed by confirmatory bacterial culture (P=.0065).[25]

Overlapping Symptoms/Clinical Presentations

The symptoms of many respiratory virus illnesses, such as fever, cough, vomiting, abdominal pain, myalgia, and headache, are often not sufficiently specific to differentiate the exact etiology for an infectious disease, and yet the treatment can vary depending on the agent. Antiviral medications are available for influenza, RSV, and severe acute respiratory syndrome coronavirus 2 (SARS-CoV-2) infections; however, the efficacy of these medications is time-sensitive, in that they are more effective when given earlier in the course of illness. In contrast, there are no antiviral medications for other respiratory viruses and treatment consists only of supportive care. Having access to molecular POC testing for these respiratory viruses can minimize the time-to-diagnosis and expedite treatment, as appropriate.

Influenza-Season Shortages

The severity of the seasonal respiratory virus, influenza, varies greatly each year. The Centers for Disease Control (CDC) estimates that influenza is responsible for 4 to 21 million medical visits in the United States alone.[26] The unpredictable surge of patients to urgent care, physician offices, and emergency departments can lead to a shortage of patient beds, health care workers, and personal protective equipment. Thus, the availability of POCT infrastructure to perform rapid, high-quality diagnostic testing can allow for shorter wait and visit times, distribute the testing across a broader network of locations, and finally, can reduce the burdens on hospitals.

CURRENT STATUS OF DIAGNOSTIC STEWARDSHIP AND POINT-OF-CARE TESTING

While diagnostic stewardship programs are not required by any US-based regulatory agencies, the CDC has incorporated a goal for the "Transatlantic task force for antimicrobial resistance," an alliance between the United States and European public health agencies, to build diagnostic stewardship as a key approach to reducing diagnostic error.[3] The CDC states that diagnostic stewardship interventions are needed in order to limit the incorrect diagnosis of infections with multidrug-resistant organisms, as well as to contribute to a more targeted and prudent use of antimicrobials. Diagnostic stewardship interventions are often built into the electronic clinical workflows and function to nudge clinicians toward better decisions. The interventions could be, for example, a simple popup that is triggered to alert the ordering provider that a test is redundant, a hard stop to prevent ordering based on institution protocols, or rules that amend reports or recommend follow-up testing based on a particular result.[27] Molecular POCT can be beneficial to patient care if used at the right time and place, and the presence of an effective diagnostic stewardship working together with antimicrobial stewardship program will play a crucial role for this to happen. However, implementing a diagnostic stewardship program for the laboratory, let alone POCT is still a work in progress for many hospital/health care systems.[28]

CHALLENGES AND STRATEGIES FOR SUCCESS FOR DIAGNOSTIC STEWARDSHIP IN THE POINT-OF-CARE SETTING

Diagnostic Stewardship is a Team Sport

Misuse of clinical testing adds unnecessary costs and can lead to incorrect diagnoses and inappropriate treatment. However, selection of the appropriate tests is becoming increasingly challenging as the number of available diagnostic tests grows.[5] Looking at lessons learned from antimicrobial stewardship programs, many studies show that rapid diagnostics only improve clinical outcomes if they are coupled with stewardship teams that properly interpret results and apply them to treatment decisions.[29–35] Diagnostic stewardship programs have been established in many inpatient settings with representation from infectious diseases physicians, infectious diseases pharmacy, medical microbiologists, and laboratory directors to help establish guidance for test utilization and to provide real-time information to the ordering clinicians.[3] However, similar programs have not been broadly established in the outpatient setting. A successful diagnostic stewardship program in the POC setting must have a similar team of individuals working to provide testing guidance and support in order to be successful. Additionally, successful hospital-based diagnostic stewardship programs are paired with antimicrobial stewardship programs with aligned goals. Antimicrobial stewardship should also be involved in diagnostic stewardship programs in the outpatient settings.

Many institutions have POC testing coordinators or equivalent who are the cornerstone of an efficiently operated POCT program.[36] POCT coordinators will also need to be brought in the diagnostic stewardship team and will play an important role. Besides their usual tasks of supporting the POCT test operation and QA/QC monitoring, they should also be educated to fully understand the task of result interpretation and consecutive action of each particular molecular POC test.

Order-Based Decision Support Tools

A major challenge with building diagnostic stewardship tools in the outpatient setting is the challenge of building decision support tools. In the hospital setting, diagnostic stewardship goals are often operationalized through tools built into electronic medical record (EMR) systems that guide clinicians to the right test. This strategy presents a unique challenge for the outpatient setting because POCT may be ordered and performed outside of EMR systems. EMR systems are used as an endpoint documentation location, but will lack the decision support tools used for other laboratory-based testing orders.

Regulatory Compliance

Clinical laboratories often have robust infrastructure to monitor the laboratory and testing for regulatory compliance. The clinical laboratory ensures that policies are in place, training is complete, and that quality controls (QC) pass as expected. The laboratory is also able to reject samples that do not meet appropriate specimen collection requirements (ie collection container or storage conditions). However, in a POC testing setting, meeting regulatory compliance can be much more challenging. While POC coordinators are often available for support to prepare documentation, train end-users, and monitor that QC is complete, typically there is no close oversight of the day-to-day operations of POC testing from laboratory personnel who have sufficient knowledge of regulatory compliance requests. Moreover, a few features of POC testing also present special challenge to regulatory compliance. Typically, POC testing operators are hospital staff to whom performing POC testing is only a small part of their routine duty which happens once in a while. It could be challenging to keep their familiarity to a particular test even with the required training and annual/semi-annual competency assessment. The resulting of POC testing could also be prone to manual entering error if the POC testing is not set up with proper information systems connectivity. Meeting the request of external QC runs at certain frequency (eg, weekly or monthly) can be problematic unless the test instrument has a locked down function.

Clinical Utility

Defining the appropriate clinical utility of single target-based molecular POC tests is generally less complex than that of a syndromic panel. However, the new availability of multiplex respiratory panels can present challenges for defining testing algorithms in POC settings. Most of the commercially-available syndromic-based respiratory panels do not allow for target customization. For this reason, multiplex panels are often strictly restricted in hospital-based settings to only test when pretest probability is moderate to high for more than 1 target on the panel, when results will influence management, or for high-risk or immunocompromised patients.[5,37] Multiple studies have shown that the availability of multiplex respiratory pathogen tests alone did not make a difference in antibiotic prescription in ED peds and adult outpatient populations.[28,38,39] Reischi and colleagues demonstrated that the use of the FA did not result in a significant reduction of antibiotic treatment or in length of hospital stay in a pediatric inpatient population.[20] In the POC setting, clear guidelines need to be implemented to guide the appropriate utilization of these panels in order to realize benefits for patient management.

Intended Use

While molecular POC testing for sexually-transmitted infections offers distinct advantages, there are several challenges that need to be addressed before they are broadly implemented. Firstly, the binx Chlamydia/Gonorrhoeae test recommends that negative male urine samples get reflexed to a clinical laboratory for additional, confirmatory testing. The urine specimen collection container for the binx test is a proprietary collection container with preservative. Either clinical laboratories will need to validate the binx collection device for use on their in-house test or the clinic would have to collect an additional specimen from the patient. It is essential that electronic infrastructure is developed in order to ensure that the appropriate samples are automatically reflexed to the clinical laboratory as needed. Developing this infrastructure will be challenging in the event that the testing is done outside of electronic medical documentation systems. Finally, clarity will be needed on the regulatory requirements for POC molecular STI testing. It is unclear if and how positive results will be reported to health agencies or if the overall test positivity rates will need to be monitored and problems investigated, as is the case in high-complexity clinical laboratories.

SUMMARY

Incorporating molecular testing into a POC setting offers distinct advantages for patient care. Timely, high-quality results at the patient bedside can expedite the time to appropriate treatment. However, there are challenges that need to be addresses before these tests are more broadly utilized. Diagnostic stewardship teams should be put into place to help guide providers on the appropriate test utilization. End users need to be educated on regulatory standards and proper pre-analytic, analytical, and post-analytic concerns for each test. Finally, electronic infrastructure as for decision support tools should be deployed to empower end users with confidence that the tests are being utilized in the appropriate settings.

CLINICS CARE POINTS

- The first CLIA-waived molecular test was approved for clinical use in 2015 for the detection of Influenza A and B. There are currently 17 CLIA-waived molecular tests on the market for infectious diseases.
- Point of care molecular tests are more sensitive than antigen tests and culture, thus enabling clinicians to make informed and timely decisions for patient care, such as discontinuing unnecessary antibiotics, initiating antiviral use, or guiding infection control decisions.
- Diagnostic stewardship programs have been shown to optimize diagnostic testing for inpatients, but these programs have not yet been implemented in point-of-care settings. Numerous barriers must be overcome before diagnostic stewardship programs can be broadly implemented for point-of-care.

REFERENCES

1. Dik JW, Poelman R, Friedrich AW, et al. An integrated stewardship model: antimicrobial, infection prevention and diagnostic (AID). Future Microbiol 2016;11(1):93–102.
2. Messacar K, Parker SK, Todd JK, et al. Implementation of rapid molecular infectious disease diagnostics: the role of diagnostic and antimicrobial stewardship. J Clin Microbiol 2017;55(3):715–23.
3. Morgan DJ, Malani PN, Diekema DJ. Diagnostic stewardship to prevent diagnostic error. JAMA 2023;329(15):1255–6.

4. Claeys KC, Johnson MD. Leveraging diagnostic stewardship within antimicrobial stewardship programmes. Drugs Context 2023;12. https://doi.org/10.7573/dic.2022-9-5.
5. Patel R, Fang FC. Diagnostic stewardship: opportunity for a laboratory-infectious diseases partnership. Clin Infect Dis 2018;67(5):799–801. https://doi.org/10.1093/cid/ciy077.
6. McGinn T, Cohen S, Khan S, et al. The high cost of low value care. Trans Am Clin Climatol Assoc 2019;130:60–70.
7. Morgan DJ, Malani P, Diekema DJ. Diagnostic stewardship-leveraging the laboratory to improve antimicrobial use. JAMA 2017;318(7):607 8.
8. Brown S, Dickerson J. The struggle is real: lab leaders discuss utilization challenges during a 2-day summit. J Appl Lab Med 2016;1(3):306–9. https://doi.org/10.1373/jalm.2016.020792.
9. (DLS) DoLS. Clinical Laboratory Improvement Amendments (CLIA) Test Complexities. Centers for Disease control. Updated August 6, 2018. Accessed 10-26-2023, 2023. https://www.cdc.gov/clia/test-complexities.html.
10. Burtis CA, Bruns DE, Sawyer BG, et al. Tietz fundamentals of clinical chemistry and molecular diagnostics. Seventh edition. Elsevier/Saunders; 2015. p. 1075, xxii.
11. Nichols JH. Utilizing point-of-care testing to optimize patient care. EJIFCC 2021;32(2):140–4.
12. Green DA, StGeorge K. Rapid antigen tests for influenza: rationale and significance of the fda reclassification. J Clin Microbiol 2018;56(10).
13. Chartrand C, Tremblay N, Renaud C, et al. Diagnostic accuracy of rapid antigen detection tests for respiratory syncytial virus infection: systematic review and meta-analysis. J Clin Microbiol 2015;53(12):3738–49.
14. Gentilotti E, De Nardo P, Cremonini E, et al. Diagnostic accuracy of point-of-care tests in acute community-acquired lower respiratory tract infections. A systematic review and meta-analysis. Clin Microbiol Infect 2022;28(1):13–22.
15. Parker KG, Gandra S, Matushek S, et al. Comparison of 3 nucleic acid amplification tests and a rapid antigen test with culture for the detection of group a streptococci from throat swabs. J Appl Lab Med 2019;4(2):164–9.
16. Claeys KC, Morgan DJ, Leekha S, et al. Diagnostic and antimicrobial stewardship with molecular respiratory testing across the SHEA Research Network. Infect Control Hosp Epidemiol 2021;42(8):1010–3.
17. Kozel TR, Burnham-Marusich AR. Point-of-Care testing for infectious diseases: past, present, and future. J Clin Microbiol 2017;55(8):2313–20.
18. Otto CC, Kaplan SE, Stiles J, et al. Rapid molecular detection and differentiation of influenza viruses A and B. J Vis Exp 2017;119. https://doi.org/10.3791/54312.
19. Nie SP, Roth RB, Stiles J, et al. Evaluation of Alere i influenza A&B for rapid detection of influenza viruses A and B. J Clin Microbiol 2014;52(9):3339–44.
20. Reischl AT, Schreiner D, Poplawska K, et al. The clinical impact of PCR-based point-of-care diagnostic in respiratory tract infections in children. J Clin Lab Anal 2020;34(5):e23203.
21. Van Der Pol B, Taylor SN, Mena L, et al. Evaluation of the performance of a point-of-care test for Chlamydia and gonorrhea. JAMA Netw Open 2020;3(5):e204819.
22. Administration UFD. Devices@FDA. Accessed 10/26/2023, https://www.accessdata.fda.gov/scripts/cdrh/devicesatfda/index.cfm.
23. Shulman ST, Bisno AL, Clegg HW, et al. Clinical practice guideline for the diagnosis and management of group A streptococcal pharyngitis: 2012 update by the Infectious Diseases Society of America. Clin Infect Dis 2012;55(10):1279–82.

24. Thompson TZ, McMullen AR. Group A Streptococcus testing in pediatrics: the move to point-of-care molecular testing. J Clin Microbiol 2020;58(6).
25. Rao A, Berg B, Quezada T, et al. Diagnosis and antibiotic treatment of group a streptococcal pharyngitis in children in a primary care setting: impact of point-of-care polymerase chain reaction. BMC Pediatr 2019;19(1):24.
26. Control CfD. Influenza (Flu) Past Seasons Estimated Influenza Disease Burden. Updated October 18, 2022. Accessed 10-26-2023, 2023. https://www.cdc.gov/flu/about/burden/past-seasons.html.
27. Otto CC, Shuptar SL, Milord P, et al. Reducing unnecessary and duplicate ordering for ovum and parasite examinations and Clostridium difficile PCR in immunocompromised patients by using an alert at the time of request in the order management system. J Clin Microbiol 2015;53(8):2745–8.
28. Mattila S, Paalanne N, Honkila M, et al. Effect of point-of-care testing for respiratory pathogens on antibiotic use in children: a randomized clinical trial. JAMA Netw Open 2022;5(6):e2216162.
29. Bauer KA, West JE, Balada-Llasat JM, et al. An antimicrobial stewardship program's impact with rapid polymerase chain reaction methicillin-resistant Staphylococcus aureus/S. aureus blood culture test in patients with S. aureus bacteremia. Clin Infect Dis 2010;51(9):1074–80.
30. Huang AM, Newton D, Kunapuli A, et al. Impact of rapid organism identification via matrix-assisted laser desorption/ionization time-of-flight combined with antimicrobial stewardship team intervention in adult patients with bacteremia and candidemia. Clin Infect Dis 2013;57(9):1237–45.
31. Bauer KA, Perez KK, Forrest GN, et al. Review of rapid diagnostic tests used by antimicrobial stewardship programs. Clin Infect Dis 2014;59(Suppl 3):S134–45.
32. Perez KK, Olsen RJ, Musick WL, et al. Integrating rapid diagnostics and antimicrobial stewardship improves outcomes in patients with antibiotic-resistant Gram-negative bacteremia. J Infect 2014;69(3):216–25.
33. Banerjee R, Teng CB, Cunningham SA, et al. Randomized trial of rapid multiplex polymerase chain reaction-based blood culture identification and susceptibility testing. Clin Infect Dis 2015;61(7):1071–80.
34. Lockwood AM, Perez KK, Musick WL, et al. Integrating rapid diagnostics and antimicrobial stewardship in two community hospitals improved process measures and antibiotic adjustment time. Infect Control Hosp Epidemiol 2016;37(4):425–32.
35. Minejima E, Wong-Beringer A. Implementation of rapid diagnostics with antimicrobial stewardship. Expert Rev Anti Infect Ther 2016;14(11):1065–75.
36. Gledhill TR, White SK, Lewis JE, et al. A profile of point of care coordinators: roles, responsibilities and attitudes. Lab Med 2019;50(3):e50–5.
37. Ramanan P, Bryson AL, Binnicker MJ, et al. Syndromic panel-based testing in clinical microbiology. Clin Microbiol Rev 2018;31(1).
38. Green DA, Hitoaliaj L, Kotansky B, et al. Clinical utility of on-demand multiplex respiratory pathogen testing among adult outpatients. J Clin Microbiol 2016;54(12):2950–5.
39. Velly L, Cancella de Abreu M, Boutolleau D, et al. Point-of-care multiplex molecular diagnosis coupled with procalcitonin-guided algorithm for antibiotic stewardship in lower respiratory tract infection: a randomized controlled trial. Clin Microbiol Infect 2023. https://doi.org/10.1016/j.cmi.2023.07.031.

Preanalytical Challenges of Molecular Microbiology Tests

Anisha Misra, PhD[a], Eleanor A. Powell, PhD[b,*]

KEYWORDS

- Preanalytical • Specimen type • DNA/RNA storage • Specimen processing
- Specimen collection device

KEY POINTS

- Molecular testing may allow for less-invasive specimen types to be used than culture-based testing but data vary by specimen type and pathogen.
- Specimen containers must be free from contaminating nucleic acids and from substances that may inhibit amplification.
- Proper specimen transport and storage conditions are essential to ensure nucleic acids are not degraded.

INTRODUCTION

One of the most common sayings in laboratory medicine is "garbage in, garbage out." This saying highlights the importance of preanalytical factors when considering overall result quality. Minimizing preanalytical errors is key to a laboratory quality assurance program because approximately 46% to 68.2% of all laboratory errors occur in the preanalytical phase.[1] For infectious disease testing, preanalytical issues have traditionally been concerned with ensuring adequate sampling and maintaining organism viability. Because molecular methods play an increasingly large role in microbiology diagnostics, maintaining organism viability may be less important but specimens must be free of not only contaminating organisms but also contaminating nucleic acids. Furthermore, the increased sensitivity of many molecular methods as compared with culture may redefine "adequate" sampling, allowing less-invasive specimen types to be used.

[a] Department of Laboratory Medicine, Cleveland Clinic, Robert J. Tomsich Pathology and Laboratory Medicine Institute, 10300 Carnegie Avenue LL-1, Cleveland, OH 44195, USA; [b] Department of Pathology and Laboratory Medicine, University of Cincinnati College of Medicine, 3188 Bellevue Avenue, Cincinnati, OH 45219, USA

* Corresponding author.

E-mail address: powelleo@ucmail.uc.edu

Clin Lab Med 44 (2024) 33–43
https://doi.org/10.1016/j.cll.2023.10.007

Many of these preanalytical issues were highlighted and debated during the early days of the coronavirus disease 2019 (COVID-19) pandemic. Are nasal swabs sensitive enough for COVID-19 testing or are nasopharyngeal (NP) swabs required? Are bronchoalveolar lavages (BALs) required for critically ill patients? Can saline be used instead of viral transport media? Is any sort of transport media even required? For how long are specimens stable? Do they need to be frozen immediately or will a freeze–thaw cycle reduce sensitivity?

In this review, we will explore some of the preanalytical factors that may pose challenges for molecular testing, including specimen type selection, specimen collection procedures, specimen collection devices, storage and transport conditions, and specimen-processing procedures.

DISCUSSION

Specimen Type

When selecting which specimen type should be used for molecular testing, it is necessary to weigh the benefits of maximizing test sensitivity and specificity with considerations such as patient comfort, patient acceptance, and the risks and costs of acquiring more invasive specimens. Although this balance is both pathogen-specific and patient-specific, data are available for a variety of body systems.

Upper respiratory infections

One of the key questions of the early COVID-19 pandemic was which specimens were optimal and which specimens were acceptable. Although this was highlighted by the pandemic, similar questions have been investigated for other upper respiratory infections. Traditionally NP swabs have been the specimen of choice for upper respiratory infections but these require trained collectors, and they can be painful for and poorly received by patients. For culture-based influenza testing, using a nasal swab resulted in decreased sensitivity as compared with an NP swabs (40% vs 51%) but this difference was decreased when molecular methods were used.[2] Similarly, detection of adenovirus, respiratory syncytial virus (RSV), parainfluenza, and influenza viruses were detected at lower rates in nasal swabs when compared with NP aspirates (a common alternative to NP swabs for small children) when viral culture or immunofluorescence were used; when polymerase chain reaction (PCR) was used, diagnostic yields were similar for all viruses except RSV.[3] A literature review of studies examining influenza specimen types for PCR-based testing found that 2 combined less-invasive specimens (such as oropharyngeal and nasal swabs) had similar sensitivity to NP swabs in adults, and in children, there were no statistical differences in sensitivity among NP swabs, NP washes, NP aspirates, oropharyngeal swabs, or nasal swabs.[4] For severe acute respiratory syndrome coronavirus 2 (SARS-CoV-2), a metanalysis using NP swabs as the gold standard also found that combined nasal and oropharyngeal swabs had equivalent sensitivity to NP swabs but nasal swabs alone and saliva also had acceptable sensitivity, whereas oropharyngeal swabs did not.[5] Although age-related stratification typically focuses on children, there is some evidence that oropharyngeal swabs may not be ideal for people aged older than 60 years because respiratory pathogen viral loads were 19 times higher in the nasopharynx than the oropharynx in this population.[6]

Using less-invasive specimen types is preferred by patients. When comparing NP swabs and nasal washes, 91% of patients preferred the nasal wash experience, and clinical sensitivity was not affected.[7] Similarly, patients reported equivalent discomfort with nasal aspirates, nasal washes, and nasal swabs.[8] Using less-invasive specimen types (such as nasal swabs or saliva) also allows for self-collection without losing sensitivity, even when collection is not observed by a health-care provider.[9,10]

Lower respiratory infections

Although many studies have examined how specimen type affects sensitivity for molecular diagnostics of upper respiratory infections, very little data are available for lower respiratory tract specimens. Data from culture-based testing shows a high concordance between sputum culture and BAL fluids culture (93.7% of specimens collected within 1 day of the other and 96.5% within 7 days), although BALs may increase sensitivity when diagnosing hospital-acquired pneumonia.[11,12] Studies comparing specimen types for molecular methods have focused on *Mycobacterium tuberculosis* (MTB) and *Pneumocystis jirovecii* (PJP). One study performed MTB PCR on paired sputum and BAL specimens from 258 patients with smear-negative MTB infections.[13] PCR on BAL specimens was more sensitive than when sputum specimens were tested (41.9% vs 32.1%) but testing both specimens resulted in the greatest diagnostic yield (62.8% sensitive). Similarly, testing BAL specimens was more sensitive than sputum when performing PCR for PJP in immunocompromised patients (100% vs 86.6%).[14] One study explored specimen type differences when using metagenomic next-generation sequencing (mNGS).[15] In this study, BAL and sputum specimens were collected from 32 patients, and both specimens underwent mNGS. There were no differences in sensitivity or specificity between specimen types when comparing results to culture. Further studies are needed to fully elucidate potential differences in performance of different specimen types for molecular diagnostics of lower respiratory infections. As a Food and Drug Administration (FDA)-approved multiplex PCR panel is now available for use on both invasive and noninvasive lower respiratory specimens, such studies will help maximize diagnostic yield while minimizing patient risk and discomfort.[16]

Sexually transmitted infections

For Sexually transmitted infection (STI) diagnostics, there is a strong trend toward less invasive or self-collected specimens. Because these may not require a genital or pelvic examination, patients may be more likely to consent, and collection can occur at locations more convenient for patients, including their home.[17,18] For STI testing in women, endocervical swabs have traditionally been the preferred specimen because other specimens resulted in unacceptable sensitivity for *Neisseria gonorrhoeae* (NG) culture.[19] When molecular methods are used, vaginal swabs are noninferior to endocervical swabs for *Chlamydia trachomatis* (CT) and NG testing.[20] Although urine was the preferred sample type among surveyed patients, a metanalysis found that vaginal swabs had superior sensitivity (96.5% in vaginal swabs vs 90.7% in urine for NG; 94.1% in vaginal swabs vs 86.9% in urine for CT).[18,21] The study found that for *Trichomonas vaginalis*, differences in sensitivity are not statistically significant, although superior sensitivity for vaginal swabs trends toward significance. For human papillomavirus (HPV), endocervical swabs are the standard specimen type used by most FDA-approved assays, likely due to the use of HPV PCR as a reflex test from abnormal Pap smears. Despite this, data from multiple studies show that vaginal swabs have equivalent sensitivity as compared with endocervical swabs, although the rate of invalid results may be higher with self-collected vaginal swabs.[19,22,23] For STI testing in men, a metanalysis found that the sensitivity of urine specimens compared with urethral swabs is 88% for CT and 92% for NG.[24] Urethral swabbing is associated with moderate-to-severe pain in patients, so despite decreased sensitivity, urine is the recommended specimen type for genital STI screening in men.[25]

Gastrointestinal disease

Bulk stool has been the specimen historically used for bacterial enteric pathogen culture, although rectal swabs may be more convenient and acceptable for patients because they do not require at-home stool collection. Rectal swabs have historically been found to be less sensitive than bulk stool, although advances in swab technology have minimized this difference in recent years.[26] Studies exploring the use of gastrointestinal (GI) panels on rectal swabs have found that this is as sensitive as culture of rectal swabs and is equivalent in performance to GI panels on bulk stool.[27,28] Similarly, when using singleplex PCR for rotavirus and norovirus, performance is equivalent between bulk stool and rectal swabs.[29,30] Although gut microbiome analysis is not yet available as a clinical assay, data from several studies suggest that rectal swabs can also reliably be used instead of bulk stool for these purposes.[31–33]

Tissue infections

Molecular testing of tissue specimens is not yet widely available because there are no FDA-approved methods. Broad-range bacterial and fungal sequencing is, however, available at some references laboratories, and proper specimen selection is key to maximize diagnostic yield while minimizing nonsignificant or potentially misleading results. When considering broad-range fungal sequencing, a study found that sequencing formalin-fixed paraffin-embedded (FFPE) tissue is less sensitive than culture but sequencing fresh tissue has equivalent sensitivity.[34] Specimens from open resections had higher diagnostic yield than fine needle aspirations and biopsies. When FFPE tissue is tested, both positivity and rates of clinically relevant results were significantly higher when fungal elements were seen in pathology slides; only 3.0% of specimens yielded clinically relevant detections when fungal elements were not seen.[35] Multiple studies have found that joint tissue and cardiac tissue have the highest diagnostic yield for broad range sequencing, whereas the yield with blood specimens is low, and lower respiratory specimens are associated with high rates of clinically irrelevant detections.[36,37] Additional studies are needed to fully determine the best specimens for broad range sequencing to maximize diagnostic yield.

Specimen type summary

In general, molecular methods make using less-invasive specimen types more feasible than with culture-based methods. It is, however, important to note that there are still significant differences in sensitivity for some specimen types, so clinical judgment is required to determine the most appropriate specimen type. Using less-invasive specimen types may be of particular utility when coupled with at-home or mobile specimen collection, such as for STIs or in respiratory virus outbreaks. Additional studies will be required to determine ideal specimen types because more multiplex panels, Sanger sequencing assays, and next-generation sequencing tests are available; because these tests are significantly more expensive and more sensitive than culture-based methods, appropriate specimen type selection will be key for best diagnostic stewardship.

Specimen Collection, Transport, and Processing

Determining the appropriate specimen for testing is only half the battle. Maintaining stability of said specimen, and limiting contamination or introduction of inhibitory substances during transport and processing is imperative to molecular microbiology testing. Microbiology laboratories within each institution need to provide guidelines for clinical teams on the appropriate collection device and volume, as well as time and temperature conditions in which the specimen will remain stable until receipt into the clinical microbiology laboratory. Molecular assays are also more prone to inhibitory molecules that are endogenous to the specimen type or collection device but can also be introduced exogenously. Utilization of sterile techniques during collection and transportation of specimens, regulating shared specimens and preferring collection of microbiology-specific specimens are important preanalytical strategies to implement for molecular testing. Cumulatively, they can prevent both false-positive and false-negative results.

We will discuss the challenges of collection, transport, and handling of the specimen types discussed in the previous "Specimen Type" section. There are some general principles that apply to all molecular testing regardless of specimen type that are important to consider before diving into specifics. RNA is generally more labile than DNA due to its structure and the abundance of ribonucleases (RNases) in the environment, including in microbes.[38,39] Quality of RNA has been shown to decline as quickly as 24 hours, whereas DNA quality remained consistent even at 15 days.[40] Recently, liquid biopsy, which is based on detecting circulating cell-free DNA (cfDNA) from invasive microbes in blood has shown increased sensitivity and specificity for a variety of pathogens.[41–43] Applying best practices to preserve the integrity of nucleic acid before analysis is integral to obtaining accurate results.

Specimen Collection and Transport by Collection Containers

Anticoagulants for blood

These principles are especially highlighted when using blood and its components for molecular assays. Heparin is widely used for blood collection for a variety of tests but is historically known to be inhibitory for molecular assays.[44] There is new evidence to show that heparin may not affect amplification when large amounts of DNA are present or for intracellular RNA.[40,45] Even so, heparin is avoided as a collection container additive for molecular assays. Ethylenediaminetetraacetic acid (EDTA) and/or acid citrate dextrose are the preferred additives for blood when molecular assays need to be performed. EDTA acts as a chelating agent and prevents nucleases from degrading DNA.[46] Similarly acid citrate dextrose prevents fragmentation of DNA and RNA, yielding a higher quality specimen for molecular assays.[47] Keeping in mind the varying stability of RNA versus DNA or now cell-free RNA and/or DNA, the collection device is specific to the analyte being evaluated in the molecular assay. If intracellular RNA is being measured, collection tubes with RNA-stabilizing agents can not only prevent degradation but also limit unintended changes in gene expression.[48]

Other factors such as time until processing and storage temperatures also vary depending on the components, with the goal to keep DNA/RNA as stable as possible. Studies have shown that minimizing cell lysis has increased stability of cfDNA. For cfDNA, cellular components are isolated from liquid phase as soon as possible.[49] A metanalysis study to determine the time-point at which cfDNA levels can remain stable found varied answers. It recommends blood should be processed for cfDNA within 6 hours of collection in an EDTA tube, although the studies included within the analysis varied on stability from 0 to 24 hours when an EDTA tubed was used. Stability was extended to up to 10 days in studies when collection tube contained preservative that prevented lysis of peripheral leukocytes.[49] Freezing whole blood does not increase stability and even damages RNA but blood components such as plasma and serum can be frozen to maintain integrity.[40,50] Bone marrow can be refrigerated but needs to be processed within 72 hours. Freezing can extend stability of bone marrow sample but only if red blood cells have been removed to prevent lysis and release of heme, which inhibit molecular assays.[51] Instructions detailing the collection and storage need to be developed for all different specimen types but also considering the analyte.

Fixatives for stool

Specific transport vials and temperature conditions can increase the longevity of stool samples. Stool has abundant microbes, making it a challenging specimen for molecular assays. Fixatives are needed not only to preserve the integrity of certain pathogens but also to inhibit overgrowth of normal flora and prevent shearing of nucleic acid.

Fixatives (formalin, sodium acetate-acetic acid-formalin [SAF], and low viscosity polyvinyl alcohol [LV-PVA]) that have been developed for stool culture and/or identification of organisms by microscopy may not always be appropriate for molecular testing.[52] These fixatives may contain inhibitors that interfere with efficient extraction and amplification of nucleic acid in specimens. Fecal DNA stabilizers such as the economic 95% ethanol[53] or single vial fixatives such as Cary-blair, Totalfix, and Ecofix are needed to proceed with molecular testing.[52] These fixatives are free of inhibitors, can prevent degradation of nucleic acid even when stored long term at room temperature. Unpreserved stool, however, can negatively affect the integrity of nucleic acid. However, even more concerning is the overgrowth of commensal flora, which significantly influence the sensitivity of detection of enteropathogens by molecular tests when low pathogen burden present or due to excessive generation of inhibitory molecules.[54,55] Studies have shown that freezing stool specimens can also inhibit the growth of normal flora without affecting the quality of nucleic acid present.[56] Thus, storage temperature along with preserving stool in fixatives can increase stability of analytes in stool specimens considerably especially during transport and delays in molecular testing.[56]

Swabs

Swabs are generally not the preferred specimen in microbiology but they are ideal for collection of buccal, NP, cervical, and urethral samples. Swabs are not all made the same and are not interchangeable among the specimen types listed.[57] Cotton or wood shaft swabs are not recommended for the detection by molecular assays, as the sample can be hard to elute, and the wood shaft can absorb the elution buffer resulting in false negatives.[58] During the pandemic, however, due to the supply chain shortages, these notions were challenged, and some studies found no meaningful differences between the different swab types.[57,58] As it is so appropriately said, "desperate times, call for desperate measures." In general, dacron/nylon swabs are preferred for respiratory specimens even over synthetic rayon swabs.[57] Swabs should typically be transported in viral transport media at 4°C for a few days. If the specimen needs to be stored for longer periods, then it should be placed at −70°C for optimal recovery.[57]

STI detection has been revolutionized initially by molecular testing but also by the ease, flexibility, and privacy of self-collect specimens. Moreover, self-collection has the ability to reach the population highest at risk for STIs.[59] Ease of shipping and storage conditions are especially important for self-collect specimens. Various studies have shown that for the detection of most STIs, both dry swab and a swab shipped in liquid medium are equivalent.[60,61] Nucleic acid stability within swab collected specimens can vary by storage conditions and depends on DNA versus RNA pathogen.[50] DNA pathogens are hardier and can remain stable up to a month at room temperature for HPV, whereas respiratory viruses are stable for only 4 days at 4°C.[50] Testing specimens from swabs has always been challenging but ESwabs (Copan Diagnostics Inc., Murrieta, CA) have revolutionized specimen collection on swabs. ESwabs are a flocked swab that comes with 1 mL of Liquid Amies allowing for improved specimen collection and elution. It also standardizes the volume of specimen per collection allowing for wide use within the clinical microbiology laboratory.[62]

Specimen processing

The variable effects of transportation and storage of specimens have been discussed earlier, and although ideally specimens would be collected and processed the same day, that is not always the case. It becomes important to not only maintain optimal storage conditions during transport but beyond that and to perform testing before stability expires. It is also important to maintain sterile conditions during the extended storage period and during the initial processing of specimens. This is especially important for molecular testing due to its inherent sensitivity as compared with traditional culture methods.

Broad-range next-generation sequencing for bacterial, fungal, and mycobacterial targets can aid in diagnosis; however, any results obtained should be correlated clinically and with other pathologic findings. Next-generation sequencing is highly sensitive and relatively unbiased in its nature and thus cannot differentiate between an unlikely true pathogen and a contaminant. This is less of an issue for isolate sequencing versus direct-from-sample sequencing. Contaminating organisms can be introduced into these heterogenous tissue samples at any time point from collection, transport, processing and actual sequencing of the specimen thus it is vital to take preventative measures such as maintaining sterile techniques, unidirectional workflows, and identifying common contaminants.[63] This can be even more challenging with fungal sequencing because fungal spores are ubiquitous in the environment. In addition to engineering workflows, one has to maintain the integrity of all reagents and plastics. At the current time, companies cannot ensure reagents and plastics are not contaminated with fungal DNA.[64–66] It is important to consider contamination during the preanalytical steps to not further abrogate the issue. It is important to note, however, that contamination may be resolved using bioinformatics and clinical correlation postanalytically by setting reporting thresholds, and determining local contaminants that should never be reported.[67]

SUMMARY

Because the clinical microbiology laboratories use more molecular testing, it is important to have guard rails for the preanalytical steps that can have significant impact on patient test results. Understanding preanalytical factors can maximize result quality while minimizing patient discomfort, invalid results, the need for recollections, and irrelevant or contaminated results. With the advent of more and more laboratory-developed molecular tests, it is important to evaluate the preanalytical steps for the specimen collection, transport, storage, and processing in addition to analytical performance. Placing strict and detailed acceptability criteria for these diagnostic assays is essential for accuracy and quality of results.

CLINICS CARE POINTS

- Less-invasive specimen types have generally acceptable sensitivity when testing for upper respiratory infections, STIs, and GI infections but not all specimen types will be approved for use with all assays. Clinicians should collaborate with clinical laboratorians to select appropriate specimen types when needed.
- For direct-from-specimen sequencing, preliminary studies show diagnostic yield is highest when pathogens are visible on pathology and on cardiac and joint specimens. Further studies are needed to determine ideal specimen types for metagenomic sequencing.
- Collection devices and fixatives, in general, are used to increase stability of a specimen but must be selected on careful review of the analyte to be measured. Analyte and collected device combination determine ideal storage temperature and conditions and need to be carefully optimized.

- Exogenous introduction of contaminants is a larger problem for more sensitive assays such as molecular testing and increased rigor is needed to ensure reagents and plastics are free of nucleic acid for molecular processing.

DISCLOSURE

A. Misra has no disclosures. E.A. Powell has received research funding from GenMark Diagnostics.

REFERENCES

1. Plebani M. Errors in clinical laboratories or errors in laboratory medicine? Clin Chem Lab Med 2006;44(6):750–9.
2. Irving SA, Vandermause MF, Shay DK, et al. Comparison of nasal and nasopharyngeal swabs for influenza detection in adults. Clin Med Res 2012;10(4):215–8.
3. Sung RY, Chan PK, Choi KC, et al. A comparative study of nasopharyngeal aspirate and nasal swab specimens for the diagnosis of acute viral respiratory infection. Hong Kong Med J 2009;15(3 Suppl 4):24–7.
4. Spencer S, Thompson MG, Flannery B, et al. Comparison of respiratory specimen collection methods for detection of influenza virus infection by reverse transcription-PCR: a literature review. J Clin Microbiol 2019;57(9). https://doi.org/10.1128/JCM.00027-19.
5. Tsang NNY, So HC, Ng KY, et al. Diagnostic performance of different sampling approaches for SARS-CoV-2 RT-PCR testing: a systematic review and meta-analysis. Lancet Infect Dis 2021;21(9):1233–45.
6. Hernes SS, Quarsten H, Hagen E, et al. Swabbing for respiratory viral infections in older patients: a comparison of rayon and nylon flocked swabs. Eur J Clin Microbiol Infect Dis 2011;30(2):159–65.
7. Flynn MF, Kelly M, Dooley JSG. Nasopharyngeal swabs vs. Nasal aspirates for respiratory virus detection: a systematic review. Pathogens 2021;10(11). https://doi.org/10.3390/pathogens10111515.
8. Spyridaki IS, Christodoulou I, de Beer L, et al. Comparison of four nasal sampling methods for the detection of viral pathogens by RT-PCR-A GA(2)LEN project. J Virol Methods 2009;156(1–2):102–6.
9. Mannan N, Raihan R, Parvin US, et al. Detection of SARS-CoV-2 RNA by reverse transcription-polymerase chain reaction (RT-PCR) on self-collected nasal swab compared with professionally collected nasopharyngeal swab. Cureus 2022;14(6):e25618.
10. Kagan RM, Rogers AA, Borillo GA, et al. Performance of unobserved self-collected nasal swabs for detection of SARS-CoV-2 by RT-PCR utilizing a remote specimen collection strategy. Open Forum Infect Dis 2021;8(4):ofab039.
11. Dubourg G, Abat C, Rolain JM, et al. Correlation between sputum and bronchoalveolar lavage fluid cultures. J Clin Microbiol 2015;53(3):994–6.
12. Ranzani OT, Senussi T, Idone F, et al. Invasive and non-invasive diagnostic approaches for microbiological diagnosis of hospital-acquired pneumonia. Crit Care 2019;23(1):51.
13. Fan L, Li D, Zhang S, et al. Parallel tests using culture, xpert MTB/RIF, and SAT-TB in sputum plus bronchial alveolar lavage fluid significantly increase diagnostic performance of smear-negative pulmonary tuberculosis. Front Microbiol 2018;9:1107.

14. Pinlaor S, Mootsikapun P, Pinlaor P, et al. PCR diagnosis of Pneumocystis carinii on sputum and bronchoalveolar lavage samples in immuno-compromised patients. Parasitol Res 2004;94(3):213–8.
15. Shi W, Zhu S. The application of metagenomic next-generation sequencing in detection of pathogen in bronchoalveolar lavage fluid and sputum samples of patients with pulmonary infection. Comput Math Methods Med 2021;2021:7238495.
16. Ginocchio CC, Garcia-Mondragon C, Mauerhofer B, et al. Multinational evaluation of the BioFire(R) FilmArray(R) Pneumonia plus Panel as compared to standard of care testing. Eur J Clin Microbiol Infect Dis 2021;40(8):1609–22.
17. Chow K, Edi R, Gin G, et al. Attitudes of women participating in a clinical trial on point-of-care testing and home testing for STIs. Int J STD AIDS 2020;31(14): 1352–8.
18. Keizur EM, Bristow CC, Baik Y, et al. Knowledge and testing preferences for Chlamydia trachomatis, Neisseria gonorrhoeae, and Trichomonas vaginalis infections among female undergraduate students. J Am Coll Health 2020;68(7):754–61.
19. Coorevits L, Traen A, Binge L, et al. Identifying a consensus sample type to test for Chlamydia trachomatis, Neisseria gonorrhoeae, Mycoplasma genitalium, Trichomonas vaginalis and human papillomavirus. Clin Microbiol Infect 2018; 24(12):1328–32.
20. Krause A, Miller JB, Samuel L, et al. Vaginal swabs are non-inferior to endocervical swabs for sexually transmitted infection testing in the emergency department. West J Emerg Med 2022;23(3):408–11.
21. Aaron KJ, Griner S, Footman A, et al. Vaginal swab vs urine for detection of chlamydia trachomatis, neisseria gonorrhoeae, and trichomonas vaginalis: a meta-analysis. Ann Fam Med 2023;21(2):172–9.
22. Coorevits L, Traen A, Binge L, et al. Are vaginal swabs comparable to cervical smears for human papillomavirus DNA testing? J Gynecol Oncol 2018;29(1):e8.
23. Saville M, Hawkes D, Keung M, et al. Analytical performance of HPV assays on vaginal self-collected vs practitioner-collected cervical samples: the SCoPE study. J Clin Virol 2020;127:104375.
24. Lunny C, Taylor D, Hoang L, et al. Self-collected versus clinician-collected sampling for chlamydia and gonorrhea screening: a systemic review and meta-analysis. PLoS One 2015;10(7):e0132776.
25. Apoola A, Herrero-Diaz M, FitzHugh E, et al. A randomised controlled trial to assess pain with urethral swabs. Sex Transm Infect 2011;87(2):110–3.
26. Jean S, Yarbrough ML, Anderson NW, et al. Culture of rectal swab specimens for enteric bacterial pathogens decreases time to test result while preserving assay sensitivity compared to bulk fecal specimens. J Clin Microbiol 2019;57(6). https://doi.org/10.1128/jcm.02077-18.
27. Walker CR, Lechiile K, Mokomane M, et al. Evaluation of anatomically designed flocked rectal swabs for use with the biofire filmarray gastrointestinal panel for detection of enteric pathogens in children admitted to hospital with severe gastroenteritis. J Clin Microbiol 2019;57(12). https://doi.org/10.1128/jcm.00962-19.
28. DeBurger B, Hanna S, Powell EA, et al. Utilizing BD MAX™ enteric bacterial panel to detect stool pathogens from rectal swabs. BMC Clin Pathol 2017;17:7.
29. Sidler JA, Käch R, Noppen C, et al. Rectal swab for detection of norovirus by real-time PCR: similar sensitivity compared to faecal specimens. Clin Microbiol Infect 2014;20(12):O1017–9.
30. Gibory M, Haltbakk I, Flem E, et al. Rotavirus detection in bulk stool and rectal swab specimens in children with acute gastroenteritis in Norway. J Clin Virol 2017;97:50–3.

31. Turner G, O'Grady M, Hudson D, et al. Rectal swabs are a reliable method of assessing the colonic microbiome. Int J Med Microbiol 2022;312(2):151549.
32. Zhang N, Li TZ, Zheng K, et al. Use of rectal swab samples for analysis of the intestinal microbiome in children. Chin Med J (Engl) 2018;131(4):492–4.
33. Radhakrishnan ST, Gallagher KI, Mullish BH, et al. Rectal swabs as a viable alternative to faecal sampling for the analysis of gut microbiota functionality and composition. Sci Rep 2023;13(1):493.
34. Gomez CA, Budvytiene I, Zemek AJ, et al. Performance of targeted fungal sequencing for culture-independent diagnosis of invasive fungal disease. Clin Infect Dis 2017;65(12):2035–41.
35. Sparks R, Halliday CL, Green W, et al. Panfungal PCR on formalin-fixed, paraffin-embedded tissue: to proceed or not proceed? Pathology 2023;55(5):669–72.
36. Tkadlec J, Peckova M, Sramkova L, et al. The use of broad-range bacterial PCR in the diagnosis of infectious diseases: a prospective cohort study. Clin Microbiol Infect 2019;25(6):747–52.
37. Naureckas Li C, Nakamura MM. Utility of broad-range PCR sequencing for infectious diseases clinical decision making: a pediatric center experience. J Clin Microbiol 2022;60(5):e0243721.
38. Tan SC, Yiap BC. DNA, RNA, and protein extraction: the past and the present. J Biomed Biotechnol 2009;2009:574398.
39. Buckingham L, Flaws ML. Molecular diagnostics: fundamentals, methods, & clinical applications. Philadelphia, PA: F.A. Davis; 2007.
40. Huang LH, Lin PH, Tsai KW, et al. The effects of storage temperature and duration of blood samples on DNA and RNA qualities. PLoS One 2017;12(9):e0184692.
41. Hong DK, Blauwkamp TA, Kertesz M, et al. Liquid biopsy for infectious diseases: sequencing of cell-free plasma to detect pathogen DNA in patients with invasive fungal disease. Diagn Microbiol Infect Dis 2018;92(3):210–3.
42. Fernandez-Carballo BL, Broger T, Wyss R, et al. Toward the development of a circulating free dna-based in vitro diagnostic test for infectious diseases: a review of evidence for tuberculosis. J Clin Microbiol 2019;57(4). https://doi.org/10.1128/JCM.01234-18.
43. Long Y, Zhang Y, Gong Y, et al. Diagnosis of sepsis with cell-free DNA by next-generation sequencing technology in ICU patients. Arch Med Res 2016;47(5):365–71.
44. Satsangi J, Jewell DP, Welsh K, et al. Effect of heparin on polymerase chain reaction. Lancet 1994;343(8911):1509–10.
45. Neumaier M, Braun A, Wagener C. Fundamentals of quality assessment of molecular amplification methods in clinical diagnostics. international federation of clinical chemistry scientific division committee on molecular biology techniques. Clin Chem 1998;44(1):12–26.
46. Barra GB, Santa Rita TH, de Almeida Vasques J, et al. EDTA-mediated inhibition of DNases protects circulating cell-free DNA from ex vivo degradation in blood samples. Clin Biochem 2015;48(15):976–81.
47. Holodniy M, Mole L, Yen-Lieberman B, et al. Comparative stabilities of quantitative human immunodeficiency virus RNA in plasma from samples collected in VACUTAINER CPT, VACUTAINER PPT, and standard VACUTAINER tubes. J Clin Microbiol 1995;33(6):1562–6.
48. Stellino C, Hamot G, Bellora C, et al. Preanalytical robustness of blood collection tubes with RNA stabilizers. Clin Chem Lab Med 2019;57(10):1522–9.

49. Trigg RM, Martinson LJ, Parpart-Li S, et al. Factors that influence quality and yield of circulating-free DNA: a systematic review of the methodology literature. Heliyon 2018;4(7):e00699.
50. Sotoudeh Anvari M, Gharib A, Abolhasani M, et al. Pre-analytical practices in the molecular diagnostic tests, a concise review. Iran J Pathol. Winter 2021;16(1):1–19.
51. Akane A, Matsubara K, Nakamura H, et al. Identification of the heme compound copurified with deoxyribonucleic acid (DNA) from bloodstains, a major inhibitor of polymerase chain reaction (PCR) amplification. J Forensic Sci 1994;39(2):362–72.
52. Mathison BA, Kohan JL, Walker JF, et al. Detection of intestinal protozoa in trichrome-stained stool specimens by use of a deep convolutional neural network. J Clin Microbiol 2020;58(6). https://doi.org/10.1128/JCM.02053-19.
53. Song SJ, Amir A, Metcalf JL, et al. Preservation methods differ in fecal microbiome stability, affecting suitability for field studies. mSystems 2016;1(3). https://doi.org/10.1128/mSystems.00021-16.
54. Goneau LW, Mazzulli A, Trimi X, et al. Evaluating the preservation and isolation of stool pathogens using the COPAN fecalswab transport system and walk-away specimen processor. Diagn Microbiol Infect Dis 2019;94(1):15–21.
55. Rolhion N, Chassaing B. When pathogenic bacteria meet the intestinal microbiota. Philos Trans R Soc Lond B Biol Sci 2016;371(1707). https://doi.org/10.1098/rstb.2015.0504.
56. Choo JM, Leong LE, Rogers GB. Sample storage conditions significantly influence faecal microbiome profiles. Sci Rep 2015;5:16350.
57. Druce J, Garcia K, Tran T, et al. Evaluation of swabs, transport media, and specimen transport conditions for optimal detection of viruses by PCR. J Clin Microbiol 2012;50(3):1064–5.
58. Garnett L, Bello A, Tran KN, et al. Comparison analysis of different swabs and transport mediums suitable for SARS-CoV-2 testing following shortages. J Virol Methods 2020;285:113947.
59. Gaydos CA. Let's take a "selfie": self-collected samples for sexually transmitted infections. Sex Transm Dis 2018;45(4):278–9.
60. Gaydos CA, Crotchfelt KA, Shah N, et al. Evaluation of dry and wet transported intravaginal swabs in detection of Chlamydia trachomatis and Neisseria gonorrhoeae infections in female soldiers by PCR. J Clin Microbiol 2002;40(3):758–61.
61. Lin CQ, Zeng X, Cui JF, et al. Stability study of cervical specimens collected by swab and stored dry followed by human papillomavirus DNA detection using the cobas 4800 test. J Clin Microbiol 2017;55(2):568–73.
62. Silbert S, Kubasek C, Uy D, et al. Comparison of ESwab with traditional swabs for detection of methicillin-resistant Staphylococcus aureus using two different walk-away commercial real-time PCR methods. J Clin Microbiol 2014;52(7):2641–3.
63. Laurence M, Hatzis C, Brash DE. Common contaminants in next-generation sequencing that hinder discovery of low-abundance microbes. PLoS One 2014;9(5):e97876.
64. Czurda S, Lion T. Prerequisites for control of contamination in fungal diagnosis. Methods Mol Biol 2017;1508:249–55.
65. Czurda S, Smelik S, Preuner-Stix S, et al. Occurrence of fungal DNA contamination in PCR reagents: approaches to control and decontamination. J Clin Microbiol 2016;54(1):148–52.
66. Harrison E, Stalhberger T, Whelan R, et al. Aspergillus DNA contamination in blood collection tubes. Diagn Microbiol Infect Dis 2010;67(4):392–4.
67. Wilson MR, Sample HA, Zorn KC, et al. Clinical metagenomic sequencing for diagnosis of meningitis and encephalitis. N Engl J Med 2019;380(24):2327–40.

Diagnostic Stewardship for Multiplex Respiratory Testing

What We Know and What Needs to Be Done

Jose Lucar, MD[a], Rebecca Yee, PhD[b,*]

KEYWORDS

• Syndromic panels • Respiratory infections • Pneumonia • Diagnostic stewardship • Antimicrobial resistance • Clinical utility

KEY POINTS

- Multiplex syndromic panels can rapidly diagnose infections and detect antimicrobial resistance genes allowing for more rapid therapeutic optimization.
- Randomized controlled trials evaluating respiratory and pneumonia syndromic panels in a variety of clinical settings have generated mixed results regarding the clinical utility suggested by observational studies.
- Employing diagnostic stewardship interventions to improve appropriate clinician ordering, test interpretation, as well as laboratory specimen processing, testing, and reporting can increase clinical utility.
- Stakeholders including laboratory, antimicrobial stewardship programs, clinical end users, hospital leadership, infection prevention specialists, and information and technology specialists need to be involved in active diagnostic stewardship.

INTRODUCTION

Every year, respiratory infections are a leading cause of disease and account for many medical visits. While most respiratory illnesses are caused by viral etiologies, pneumonia can be caused by various pathogens, including bacteria, viruses, and fungi. Laboratory diagnosis of respiratory infections includes a combination of routine bacterial, fungal, and mycobacteriology cultures from respiratory specimens. Viral

[a] Division of Infectious Diseases, George Washington University School of Medicine and Health Sciences, 2150 Pennsylvania Avenue Northeast, Washington, DC 20037, USA; [b] Department of Pathology, George Washington University School of Medicine and Health Sciences, 900 23rd Street Northwest, Washington, DC 20037, USA
* Corresponding author.
E-mail address: ryee@mfa.gwu.edu

Clin Lab Med 44 (2024) 45–61
https://doi.org/10.1016/j.cll.2023.10.001

cultures that attempt to grow and identify viruses are also available although now seldom used due to long turnaround times and expertise and facility requirements needed by the laboratory. Other laboratory approaches involve immunologic assays such as direct fluorescence antibody (DFA) testing , indirect fluorescence antibody (IFA) testing, and enzyme immunoassays that detect specimen antigenic proteins on the surface of pathogens, as well as serologic tests that detect antibodies produced by the human host against a specific pathogen.

More recently, the adaptation of molecular methods such as polymerase chain reaction (PCR) has revolutionized the etiologic diagnosis of infectious diseases. There are several US Food and Drug Administration (FDA)–approved multiplex PCR panels for the detection of pathogens causing upper (>12 targets consisting of bacterial, atypical, and viral targets) as well as lower respiratory infections such as pneumonia (>15 targets consisting of bacterial, viral, and fungal targets plus select antimicrobial resistance [AMR] genes). Due to their high analytical sensitivity and short turnaround time, syndromic respiratory panels can increase the likelihood of establishing a prompt etiologic diagnosis for patients presenting with respiratory infections and have the potential to enable a more appropriate antimicrobial treatment strategy. Other benefits include support for clinical decision-making in areas such as admission, isolation, and the need for additional workup.[1,2]

Approaches to optimal implementation of syndromic respiratory panels remain unclear as there are several potential drawbacks associated with their use.[3] First, detection of an organism's nucleic acid in a multiplex PCR panel does not necessarily represent the etiologic diagnosis, while prolonged shedding of viral particles after symptoms have resolved is common. Second, detection of a viral pathogen does not exclude the possibility of bacterial coinfection. Third, a sizable number of patients that undergo syndromic respiratory panel testing have multiple targets detected at once, and interpreting these results can be a challenge for clinicians. Fourth, results from an upper respiratory panel may not correlate with the etiology of a lower respiratory tract (LRT) infection. Fifth, syndromic panels are associated with a hefty cost despite the uncertain impact on relevant health outcomes. And finally, most respiratory viruses detected in syndromic panels do not have targeted antiviral therapies available, and clinicians often do not change treatment plans based on results. With such caveats in mind, reducing diagnostic error includes the concept of overdiagnosis (ie, inability to distinguish colonization from infection) and overtreatment (ie, unnecessary workup and antibiotic therapy). Therefore, diagnostic stewardship is paramount for maximum clinical utility of these panels and can be summarized as ordering the right tests for the right patient at the right time to correctly inform clinical decision-making.

Stakeholders beyond the laboratory and antimicrobial stewardship programs (ASPs) need to be involved in various stages of the diagnostic stewardship process, including information and technology specialists, hospital leadership, end users (ie, clinicians and nurses), and infection prevention specialists. Recently, the Society for Health care Epidemiology of America convened a Diagnostic Stewardship Task Force to develop a position paper on further development of the diagnostic pathway conceptual model, including the following steps: clinician testing decision and interpretation, test ordering, specimen collection and transport to the laboratory, test processing and performance, and test reporting.[4] In this article, we will follow the diagnostic pathway conceptual model as we review the available evidence related to the optimal use of syndromic respiratory panels.

UPPER RESPIRATORY PANELS

Clinician Testing Decision, Ordering, and Achieving Actionable Outcomes: What We Know

In the context of individual patient care, testing with multiplex respiratory PCR panels (RVP) is restricted to symptomatic patients as studies have demonstrated virus shedding in asymptomatic hosts. Consecutive studies performed in adults visiting a New York City tourist attraction found that at least half of the samples were positive in asymptomatic individuals.[5,6] Positive samples included human rhinovirus, non-severe acute respiratory syndrome (SARS) coronaviruses, influenza virus, respiratory syncytial virus (RSV), and parainfluenza virus. The authors did find, however, that having symptoms was predictive of testing positive among this ambulatory adult population. Additionally, in a case-control study of children, 72% of symptomatic patients but also 35% of the asymptomatic controls tested positive for respiratory viruses, particularly for rhinovirus/enterovirus.[7] These findings highlight that results from RVP must be interpreted with caution due to high detection rates among individuals without respiratory symptoms.

In 2020, the Infectious Diseases Society of America's Diagnostics Committee (IDSA-DC) published a position statement that provided a framework for ordering molecular testing for acute respiratory tract infections which considered factors such as immunosuppression, severity of illness, underlying comorbidities, pretest probability of a given pathogen, and anticipated turnaround time to results.[8] The IDSA-DC statement highlighted that testing for viral pathogens other than influenza through RVPs is not recommended for the general pediatric and adult population presenting with an acute respiratory infection but should be considered in immunocompromised hosts and in those with severe illness. Along those lines, the American Thoracic Society published a guidance statement in 2021 addressing testing of respiratory samples for non-influenza respiratory viruses in adults with suspected community-acquired pneumonia (CAP).[9] They recommended against routine use of RVPs in the general population but suggested considering hospitalized patients with severe CAP and immunocompromised hosts while acknowledging the low quality of available evidence.

In the absence of significant risk factors for unfavorable clinical outcomes, clinical benefits from RVP testing remain mixed. There is a plethora of observational studies evaluating the potential impact of RVPs on clinical outcomes, with notable limitations and inconclusive results. Only a few prospective studies with slight clinical benefits have been published (**Table 1**). An open label, single center randomized clinical trial (RCT) found that the use of an RVP in hospitalized adults with acute LRT infection only modestly reduced the duration of intravenous antibiotics when compared with the use of routine PCR testing for common pathogens.[10] Another RCT including both children and adults presenting to an emergency department with acute LRT infection found that those tested by the RVP had fewer antibiotic prescriptions and fewer complementary studies (seen in children), with improved antiviral management of participants with influenza.[11]

In contrast, an open label, multicenter RCT conducted in adult outpatients with acute respiratory infections found that implementing an RVP did not reduce antibiotic prescription rates.[12] Another RCT evaluated adults presenting to a hospital in the United Kingdom with acute respiratory illness and fever found no difference in the proportion of patients treated with antibiotics and the mean durations of antibiotic use between both groups, though the intervention group had a shorter length of stay and improved use of antiviral treatment for those with influenza.[13] Additionally, significantly fewer patients in the multiplex PCR group received more than 1 dose of antibiotics.[13]

Table 1
Overview of studies reporting the outcomes of multiplex respiratory viral panels for upper respiratory tract infections

Population	Location	Study Design	Outcomes Impacted	Active ASP Present	Reference
Adults	Inpatients (China)	Open-label, prospective, single-center RCT	Modestly reduced the duration of intravenous antibiotics	Yes	Shengchen et al,[10] 2019
Children and adults	Emergency Department (Argentina)	Open-label, prospective, single-center RCT	Fewer antibiotic prescriptions, fewer complementary studies (in children), and improved antiviral management for influenza	Yes	Echavarría et al,[11] 2018
Adults	Outpatients (Sweden)	Open-label, prospective, multi-center RCT	No reduction in antibiotics	Not specified	Brittain-Long et al,[12] 2011
Adults	Emergency Department or Acute Medical Unit (UK)	Open-label, prospective, open-label, single-center RCT	No difference in the proportion of patients treated with antibiotics and the mean durations of antibiotic use, shorter length of stay, improved use of antiviral treatment for those with influenza	Not specified	Brendish et al,[13] 2017
Adults	Emergency Department (France)	Open-label, prospective, single-center RCT	No difference in the duration of antibiotic therapy between groups	Yes	Velly et al,[37] 2023
Adults	Inpatients (US)	Open-label, single-center RCT	No difference in antibiotic use (even with procalcitonin results), no difference in antibiotic use in hospitalized	Not specified	Branche et al,[36] 2015

Children	Inpatients (US)	Retrospective	Duration of antibiotic use shorter (in group with TAT <7 h)	Not specified	Rogers et al,[2] 2015
Adults	Emergency Department (US)	Retrospective	Reduced antibiotics in positive test admitted without radiographic findings (in group with TAT <7 h)	Yes	Weiss et al,[20] 2019
Children and Adults	Inpatient and outpatients (Turkey)	Retrospective	Higher rate of antibiotic discontinuation and lower antibiotic prescription	Yes	Keske et al,[15] 2018
Adults	Inpatients (Canada)	Retrospective	Reduction of antibiotic treatment duration with ASP	Yes	Lowe et al,[16] 2017

Abbreviations: ASP, antimicrobial stewardship program; hrs, hours; RCT, randomized controlled trial; TAT, turnaround time; UK, United Kingdom; US, United States.

In general, interventions to optimize diagnostic testing at the testing decision level include educational activities and clinician decision support tools. A recent survey of hospital epidemiology and infectious disease experts showed that nearly half of respondents did not believe that RVP improved clinical outcomes, despite other perceived benefits related to diagnosis and patient care.[14] Also, 58% of surveyed sites had implemented diagnostic stewardship to enhance the usefulness of RVPs, with education being the most common intervention (54%) but was perceived as having limited impact. Other interventions included order sets to guide test ordering, restrictions on test ordering based on clinician or patient characteristics, or structured communication of results. Along with heterogeneous prospective data assessing clinical outcomes of RVPs, the limited data on the impact of potential interventions in optimizing RVP utility have also shown mixed results.

Some retrospective interventional studies in hospitalized patients found a significantly higher rate of antibiotic discontinuation as well as an overall decrease in the total number of antibiotic prescriptions in both children and adults following implementation of the RVP plus education by the ASP.[15] An acceptance rate as high as 77% for ASP recommendations and a reduction of antibiotic treatment duration in patients with viral respiratory infections were demonstrated when there was an active targeted ASP audit and feedback.[16] However, in contrast, retrospective studies assessing the impact of real-time ASP pharmacist intervention on antibiotic de-escalation, change, or discontinuation showed that clinicians only accepted 19% to 47% of ASP recommendations.[17,18] These findings suggest that resource-intensive interventions such as direct audit-and-feedback in patients with positive RVP by trained antimicrobial stewardship providers warrant further study before widespread implementation.

Individuals presenting with an influenza-like viral illness may benefit from testing with focused molecular testing, such as influenza A/B and RSV. This includes potential candidates for antivirals during high influenza virus activity (ie, age≥65 years, history of chronic pulmonary disease, immunocompromised hosts) and patients with risk factors for complications from RSV infection (ie, history of stem cell transplant, hematologic malignancy on chemotherapy, infants<6 months). Options include primary testing for specific, single viruses (when prevalence is high) with reflex syndromic testing if initial testing is negative. Nonetheless, the American Academy of Pediatrics does not recommend RSV testing for children presenting with bronchiolitis.[19] Other variables that need to be considered include patient age, acuity of infection, vaccination status, and virus seasonality and epidemiology. Some individuals may also require testing for public health, work, or school-related reasons. Additionally, besides influenza and RSV, supportive care is typically recommended for other viral etiologies which may not warrant the need for a multiplex PCR panel, unless the test results may aid in the avoidance of unnecessary antibiotic therapy. Even in the context of SARS coronavirus 2 (SARS-CoV-2), focused molecular respiratory tests can be performed to assist in clinical decisions related to clinical interventions.

Specimen Collection, Transport, and Processing

All commercially available RVPs are validated for nasopharyngeal swabs (NPSs) (**Table 2**). NPSs are to be immediately placed into acceptable transport media, which is typically viral transport media or universal transport media but can also be in saline, M4 media, M4RT media, or into the Liquid Amies (ESwab). Specimens should be tested as soon as possible but can be refrigerated for 72 hours to 7 days and frozen at −70C for years with relatively low impact on stability. However, studies have also shown that reduced antibiotic usage and duration were seen only when test results

Table 2
Laboratory targets for diagnostic stewardship

	Upper Respiratory Viral Panel	Pneumonia Panel
Define acceptable specimens	• Nasopharyngeal swabs (manufacturer-validated) • Lower respiratory specimens (eg, BAL, sputum) if in-house validated	• BAL (including mini-BAL) • Sputum (induced, expectorated sputum, or endotracheal aspirates)
Additional concordant laboratory testing	• Not applicable	1. Gram-stains to determine sputum specimen quality. 2. Respiratory culture
Test performance concerns	• Reported low sensitivity for non–SARS-CoV-2 coronavirus, human metapneumovirus, adenovirus. Reflex testing in immunocompromised patients could be warranted. • Reported low sensitivity for atypical bacteria: *C. pneumoniae, M. pneumoniae, L. pneumophila* and *Bordetella pertussis.* Reflex testing in sputum or oropharyngeal swabs in appropriate patient population could be warranted.	• PPA and NPA varies as gold standard is culture. Molecular methods are more sensitive making difficult to distinguish non-viable cells vs colonizer vs pathogen • Low concordance rate in lower semiquantitative bins ($<10^5$ DNA copies/mL)
Test reporting	• Qualitative test: 'Detected' vs 'Not detected'	• Qualitative test: 'Detected' vs 'Not detected' • Semiquantitative bins for positive bacterial targets: 10^4, 10^5, 10^6, or $\geq 10^7$ copies/mL
Support for interpretation	• Institutional guidelines	• Provide a comment regarding semiquantitative units (in copies/mL) not being equivalent to CFU/mL • Provide a comment regarding low amounts of bacteria potentially being indicative of colonization or normal respiratory flora • Provide interpretation linking the organism and the antimicrobial susceptibility gene and therapeutic comments devised with ASP and ID teams • Institutional guidelines

(*continued on next page*)

Table 2
(continued)

	Upper Respiratory Viral Panel	Pneumonia Panel
Nudges and alerts	• Best Practice Alerts devised with ASP and IC/IP	• Best Practice Alerts devised with ASP and IC/IP
Selective reporting	• Not applicable	• Semiquantitative bins • Antimicrobial resistance genes
Framing results	• Inclusion of procalcitonin levels	• Inclusion of Gram-stain results, WBC count, and procalcitonin levels
Repeat testing	• Potential hard stop with a 10-d block • Approval with new or worsening symptoms • Testing on a BAL specimen after a negative result from NPS	

Abbreviations: ASP, antimicrobial stewardship program; BAL, bronchoalveolar lavage; CFU/mL, cell-forming units per milliliter; IC/IP, infection control and infection prevention; NPA, negative percent agreement; NPS, nasopharyngeal swabs; PPA, positive percent agreement; WBC, white blood cell.

were posted less than 7 hours after time of specimen collection suggesting that utility is greatest when testing is in-house, as opposed to being performed in reference laboratories where turnaround times can be a few days.[2,20] Some laboratories have validated the off-label use of lower respiratory specimen types such as sputum, bronchoalveolar lavage fluid samples (BAL), and bronchial washings on upper respiratory panels. Pre-processing steps such as digestion with a solution containing dithiothreitol was shown to help with specimens that originally yielded an invalid result.

Test Performance

While the overall sensitivity of RVPs is high, there are some viral targets that have slightly lower accuracy such as the non–SARS-CoV-2 coronavirus, human metapneumovirus, and adenovirus.[21,22] In immunocompromised patients, the decreased sensitivity and negative predictive value for adenovirus may miss early intervention before progression to systemic infection. Retesting negative specimens on a single-plex PCR testing showed an additional 5% increase in adenovirus cases, typically those with low viral load (Ct values >30, <106 copies/ml) and adenovirus genotypes A, D, and F.[23] The sensitivity for influenza using the BioFire FilmArray respiratory panel was greater than 73% but the updated RP.2 panel improved detection to greater than 94%.[24,25]

The other targets with variable performance are the atypical bacteria (*Chlamydia pneumoniae, Mycoplasma pneumoniae,Legionella pneumophila*) and *Bordetella pertussis*. *M pneumoniae* clinical sensitivities range from 64% to 98% depending on the platform used. The specimen type can also significantly affect clinical sensitivity.[26] Sputum was recommended for PCR detection of *M pneumoniae* by the British Thoracic Society Guidelines in 2009 after it was shown to have the highest positivity rate in a study comparing sputum, NPS, and throat swab.[27] The sensitivity for sputum versus NPS for *M pneumoniae* was 95.2% and 38.1%, respectively, whereas the specificity was 100% and 93.9%, respectively. For *C pneumoniae,* the sensitivity for sputum is greater than 95% compared to greater than 30% for NPS.[28] The sensitivity is generally greater than 80% when LRT specimens, not NPS, are tested.[29]

For detection of *B pertussis,* RVPs may use the pertussis toxin promoter target which is detected typically in highly concentrated samples (Ct value <27.0). The insertion sequence IS*481* can be used instead but IS*481* is also present in *B holmesii* and in some *B bronchiseptica*.[30] Compared to a single-plex PCR, the BioFire FilmArray RVP panel detected approximately 30% less cases.[31] In contrast, the QIAstat-DX RP assay which utilizes the IS481 insertion sequence showed 100% sensitivity in a study where the GenMark ePlex RPP assay only detected 66.7% of the specimens.[32] Hence, it is important for the clinical teams and microbiology laboratories to understand their panel targets' limitations. If clinical suspicion for atypical bacterial and/or *B pertussis* is high (eg, in pediatric populations, immunocompromised populations), a single target PCR against these targets or using a LRT specimen type may be considered for additional testing.

Laboratories may perform an off-label validation using lower respiratory specimen types on an RVP given its additional diagnostic value. Various upper RVPs can reliably detect all the targets in the BAL matrix with high precision.[33] The limit of detection (LoD) between BAL and NPS were also very comparable for viral targets; some targets even reported lower LoD in BALs.[33,34] Specificities of 100% were achieved for the targets, although false negative results with low bacterial load (CT > 30) for the atypical bacteria may also occur. However, the viscosity of the specimen could affect the sensitivity of the assay. A negative result may not necessarily rule out an infection.

Test Reporting

All the RVPs are manufactured and validated for qualitative testing. Reporting of the test results typically is either "detected" or "not detected" for each pathogen. The specimen type needs to be clearly indicated given that different clinical implications and performance characteristics may occur. Some suggest that inclusion of procalcitonin (PCT) levels into the report could help assist the clinicians in optimizing antimicrobial therapy. In a retrospective interventional study, the impact of an automated ASP electronic health record (EHR) best practice alert in inpatients with low PCT levels and a virus detected found a reduction in antibiotic use and discharge prescribing rates.[35] Meanwhile, several RCTs demonstrated that no difference in the duration of antibiotic therapy was seen when PCT levels were considered, though the standard of care group had high utilization of PCT at baseline for one of the studies.[36,37]

LOWER RESPIRATORY PANELS

Clinician Testing Decision, Ordering, and Achieving Actionable Outcomes: What We Know

A single-center prospective feasibility study evaluated the diagnostic impact of the BioFire FilmArray pneumonia panel *plus* in adults admitted with suspected CAP and found a significant reduction in the time to potentially actionable results as well as an increased microbiological yield compared with standard diagnostic microbiology methods.[38] The use of the BioFire FilmArray pneumonia panel significantly increased the detection of potential viral and bacterial pathogens in adult inpatients with CAP in another single-center prospective study.[39]

To date, there is only 1 published multicenter, randomized controlled trial evaluating the potential clinical impact of multiplex lower respiratory pneumonia PCR panels in hospitalized patients with clinical suspicion for pneumonia and risk factors for infection with gram-negative bacilli[40] (see **Table 1**). Of note, the PCR group also received active ASP recommendations approximately 5 hours after sample collection, resulting in a statistically significant reduction of 45% in inappropriate antibiotic therapy. Notably, there were no significant differences in overall antibiotic duration, the proportion of patients reaching clinical stability, length of hospital stays, rate of ICU admission, and proportion of patients being discharged from hospital. Additionally, the pneumonia PCR used in this trial showed a poor positive predictive value at 39%, a known shortcoming of these tests.

Additional data on diagnostic stewardship interventions are limited. A single-center, retrospective, preintervention and postintervention study that evaluated the impact of BioFire FilmArray pneumonia panel implementation in adult ICU patients with pneumonia was recently published.[41] That institution's pneumonia treatment guidelines recommended the use of multiplex pneumonia panel in all patients with HAP and VAP, as well as some patients with CAP (if severe, receiving broad-spectrum agents, or not improving), and the results were subject of prospective audit and feedback by their ASP. The authors found a decreasing trend (while not statistically significant) in the time to discontinuation of methicillin-resistant *Staphylococcus aureus* and antipseudomonal therapy after the implementation of the panel. It is possible that the small sample size, confounding introduced by the early months of the COVID-19 pandemic, could have impacted the results.

Specimen Collection, Transport, and Processing

Acceptable specimen types for pneumonia panels are BAL (including mini-BAL) and sputum (induced, expectorated sputum, or endotracheal aspirates) from symptomatic individuals (see **Table 2**). Specimens should be tested as soon as possible but can be stored for 1 day in 2 to 8°C. Manufacturers do not recommend specimens to be preprocessed, centrifuged, treated with any mucolytic or decontaminating agents, or placed into transport media before testing.

In general, invasive specimen types such as BAL have higher diagnostic yield than noninvasive specimens like sputum, although patients with COVID-19 have been hospitalized for pneumonia with low bacterial loads recovered in their sputum.[42] During the COVID-19 pandemic, coinfections and pneumonia were commonly seen in severely ill patients. Invasive sampling techniques were contraindicated among COVID-19 patients due to the risk of aerosol generation. That said, given the disease severity and clinical need of the patient, sputum specimens do have diagnostic advantages over BAL despite their lower yield.

Upon every lower respiratory panel request, Gram-stains are performed to determine sputum specimen quality. Typically, an acceptable sputum specimen has greater than 25 polymorphonuclear neutrophils (PMN) and less than 10 epithelial cells per high-power field (hpf) and a poor-quality specimen has greater than 25 squamous cells/hpf, and less than 25 PMN/hpf. A concomitant culture is required for organism isolation and further antimicrobial susceptibility testing.

Test Performance

Overall, the positive percent agreement (PPA) and negative percent agreement with bacterial cultures can range from 16% to 100% and 92% to 100%, respectively, with differences seen in sample types tested (eg, BAL or sputum). Instances where the panel is positive but cultures are negative may not always be interpreted as a 'false positive' since reflex testing of these same specimens using another molecular assay confirmed the original LRT panel results. At the same semi-quantification level, the concordance rate can be as low as 43% for culture-positive specimens but samples with targets detected at $\geq 10^5$ DNA copies/mL grew significantly in culture.[43] Positive predictive values of AMR genes to phenotypic antibiotic susceptibility test results range from 80% to 100%, depending on the microorganism and specific resistance marker(s).[44] The panel has excellent negative predictive value for on-panel targets. Negative results have the potential to assist in de-escalation of broad-spectrum therapy. Like RVP panels, the adenovirus target suffers from lower sensitivity. Within 6 months of the expiration date, there is a 10 to 100X loss in sensitivity for adenovirus genotype C. If there is high clinical suspicion, communication with the laboratory is necessary to ensure that the kits are not within 6 months of expiration, or another confirmatory test is recommended.

The Curetis Unyvero pneumonia panel includes *Pneumocystis jirovecii* (PJP) as a target. The PPA with standard DFA and IFA testing was 87%.[44] Studies have suggested that colonizers are more likely to have less than 10^4 copies/ml, but the panel is a qualitative test. However, the LoD of PJP on the panel is 10^5 copies/ml, so some may consider that positive detection may be associated with *P jirovecii* pneumonia.[45,46] In cases like this, reflex testing to quantitative *P jirovecii* PCR may be recommended.[47]

Test Reporting

Reporting results from pneumonia panels depends on the commercial pneumonia panel used. If the laboratory is running the Curetis Unyvero test, all targets are reported as 'detected' and 'not detected.' On the BioFire FilmArray pneumonia panel, the viral, atypical bacteria, and AMR genes are also reported as 'detected' and 'not detected.' Negative bacterial targets are reported as 'not detected' but positive bacterial targets are reported as 'detected' and in semiquantitative 'bins' of 10^4, 10^5, 10^6, or $\geq 10^7$ copies/ml.[48] However, clinical teams should not consider copies/mL as equivalent to cell-forming units (CFU)/mL, the standard quantification approach for such routine bacterial cultures as urine culture. Notating a comment in the report explaining that semiquantitative results (in copies/mL) are not equivalent to CFU/mL and may not correlate with the quantity of bacteria reported by respiratory culture may help clinical teams interpret results. Some have suggested implementing cutoffs, suppressing results from certain 'bins,' that correlate to an amount that is more commonly seen in routine culture although this would require laboratories to pursue their own validation to develop a threshold cutoff.[49]

The reports could also contain a reminder that pneumonia panels may detect low amounts of bacteria which could be indicative of colonization or normal respiratory flora, especially at institutions where there is not an active ASP. To prevent confusion in such cases, incorporating other clinical laboratory information into the same report may help clinical teams interpret the results. For example, a report could have Gram-stain result, rapid molecular result, final identification, and phenotypic susceptibility. Other strong relationships between the pneumonia panel results and true pneumonia are host inflammatory responses such as temperature (eg, fever), white blood cell count, percent polymorphonuclear lymphocytes, and PCT levels.[36,50] A benefit of combining all the results into one view is that a follow-up targeted stewardship alert can be placed to aid in the interpretation of results.

An important aspect of the pneumonia panels is the ability to detect AMR genes. Incomplete understanding of the molecular terminology can lead to ineffective treatment or missed opportunities for antimicrobial optimization. Laboratories should avoid reporting AMR results simply as 'detected' and 'not detected' without linking the organism and the AMR gene (if possible) and providing interpretation guidance.[51] It is also a College of American Pathologists requirement (checklist item MIC.21855) to link AMR determinants and phenotypic susceptibility results to a specific organism in the final patient report. For example, when *mecA* and *S aureus* are detected, proper reporting would say 'methicillin-resistant *S aureus*' or 'extended-spectrum β-lactamase (ESBL)–producing *Escherichia coli*' for an *E coli* with CTX-M gene detected. Inclusion of therapeutic comments are helpful and can be broad such as referring the team to consult the infectious diseases team, pharmacy, or specific treatment guidelines. Alternatively, the comments can contain more specific therapeutic information such as 'in the presence of a ESBL producer (CTX-M detected), a carbapenem is the drug of choice,' or 'ceftriaxone is recommended for initial therapy pending susceptibility results' (when CTX-M is not detected). Interestingly, some institutions may choose not to report the absence of CTX-M or *blaKPC* to prevent the assumptions that the organism would be susceptible to expanded-spectrum cephalosporins or carbapenems. Some laboratories only report AMR genes that are detected and suppress all 'not detected' results. Depending on your institutional and local governmental public health surveillance programs, certain drug-resistant isolates trigger isolation protocols. Laboratories should work with their antimicrobial stewardship, infection prevention, and infectious diseases teams to develop an appropriate reporting structure.

In rare cases, discrepant phenotypic and genotypic AST results may arise. Major errors defined as when an AMR gene is detected in an isolate that was susceptible to phenotypic testing or very major errors defined as when an AMR gene is not detected in an isolate found to be resistant by phenotypic testing can occur. Sometimes the AMR gene may not be detected in the organism causing the disease. Laboratories should have a process in place to resolve discordant phenotypic and genotypic susceptibility results. There are publications and resources provided by the Clinical and Laboratory Standards Institute that offer guidance to troubleshoot discrepant results.[52]

Repeat Testing

In a Centers for Medicare & Medicaid Services guidance document, repeat testing using syndromic panels with the same pathogens within 14 days for the same clinical indication is typically not covered for payment.[53] Both upper and lower respiratory panels are considered equivalent, but it must also be noted there are also less than 5 target panels that include viruses such as influenza, RSV, and SARS-CoV-2 included in the policy. Hence, it is crucial that there is judicial usage of repeat testing.

A study comparing repeat testing on NPS on both a full (>12 targets) RVP versus a smaller multiplex (<4 targets) showed that 75% of repeat tests were consistently negative, with 12% remaining positive with the same organisms upon repeat.[54] Similar findings have been reported in both adult and pediatric settings. In the immunocompromised population, especially those with concurrent symptoms like pulmonary infiltrates, fever, and hypoxia, a BAL is often performed and may include a repeat RVP. A study by Azadeh and colleagues compared the effectiveness of RVP testing on BAL samples versus NPS and found that 83% had a corresponding match in a subsequent BAL testing.[55] However, in 20% of the patients, pathogens were identified in the BAL that were not detected from the NPS. These findings indicate that once a pathogen is identified by testing NPS on RVP, subsequent testing of BAL will seldom provide new actionable clinical information. Another study performed in a bone marrow transplant pediatric population also showed that out of 140 specimens and 67 instances of repeat testing, new clinical information was only obtained in 30% of the cases and in most cases, repeat testing from an initial negative result did not change clinical management.[56] A median of 11 days elapsed between the initial and second result suggesting that a 10-day hard stop block may be a reasonable approach.[56,57] In a study with greater than 1400 specimens, savings of $140,000 per year would accrue if all repeated respiratory testing were eliminated.[54] Repeat testing may hinder clinical gain especially in cases with discordant results due to collection inadequacy. Differing results from initial runs were associated with new/

worsening symptoms and in some cases, testing on a differing specimen type such as a BAL specimen after a negative result from NPS may at times offer valuable information.

FUTURE DIRECTIONS AND SUMMARY

Many new molecular developments for multiplex testing of respiratory infections are on the horizon. At the time of writing this article, bioMérieux's SPOTFIRE respiratory panel, which consists of 15 targets, became FDA-cleared and Clinical Laboratory Improvement Amendments–waived, pioneering the introduction of molecular syndromic testing as a point of care test. For high complexity clinical laboratories, the Respiratory Pathogen ID/AMR enrichment kit (Illumina, Inc., San Diego, CA, USA), a next-generation sequencing assay developed to detect greater than 280 respiratory pathogens and AMR sequences from respiratory specimens, is also available as a laboratory-developed test. To maximize clinical utility to balance the hefty laboratory costs, respiratory panels should only ultimately be ordered if the result will affect patient management, and results should be interpreted in the clinical context. However, a strong diagnostic stewardship action plan requires robust data from research studies, preferably prospective clinical trials. Proposed areas of diagnostic stewardship research include the role of clinical decision tools (clinical decision supporting software), the impact of pairing results with clinical biomarkers, ways to enhance adherence to ASP recommendations and management guidance through EHR interventions (educational alerts, limiting test ordering according to institutional guidelines), and important health outcomes and cost-effectiveness analyses in different key populations. Diagnostic stewardship is crucial to improving patient care, but there must be a call to action for all stakeholders involved to participate in research and active implementation.

CLINICS CARE POINTS

- Multiplex syndromic upper and lower respiratory tract panels are now widely available in clinical microbiology laboratories and healthcare institutions in high resource areas.
- Observational studies have shown a potential for syndromic respiratory panels to increase the likelihood of establishing an etiological diagnosis and enabling prompt optimization of antimicrobial therapy.
- These panels have significant limitations, and evidence from prospective clinical studies have shown mixed results when evaluating actionable clinical outcomes such as reduction in inappropriate antimicrobial use, duration of therapy, and length of hospital stay.
- The approach to optimal implementation of syndromic respiratory panels remains uncertain, and further diagnostic stewardship research is needed to determine how to best use these panels to improve clinical outcomes.
- Currently, syndromic respiratory panels should only be considered in symptomatic individuals, particularly those with severe illness or immunocompromised.

DISCLOSURE

J.L reports no disclosures. R.Y. reports grants from bioMérieux, roles on committees with American Society for Microbiology, Clinical Laboratory Standards and Institutes, and Association for Molecular Pathology.

REFERENCES

1. Subramony A, Zachariah P, Krones A, et al. Impact of multiplex polymerase chain reaction testing for respiratory pathogens on healthcare resource utilization for pediatric inpatients. J Pediatr 2016;173:196–201.e2.
2. Rogers BB, Shankar P, Jerris RC, et al. Impact of a rapid respiratory panel test on patient outcomes. Archives Pathol Lab Med 2015;139(5):636–41.
3. Lewinski MA, Alby K, Babady NE, et al. Exploring the utility of multiplex infectious disease Panel Testing for diagnosis of infection in different Body sites: a Joint report of the association for molecular Pathology, American Society for microbiology, infectious diseases Society of America, and Pan American Society for clinical Virology. J Mol Diag 2023. https://doi.org/10.1016/j.jmoldx.2023.08.005. S1525-1578(23)00209-X.
4. Fabre V, Davis A, Diekema DJ, et al. Principles of diagnostic stewardship: a practical guide from the Society for healthcare epidemiology of America diagnostic stewardship Task Force. Infect Control Hosp Epidemiol 2023;44(2):178–85.
5. Shaman J, Morita H, Birger R, et al. Asymptomatic Summertime shedding of respiratory viruses. J Infect Dis 2018;217(7):1074–7.
6. Birger R, Morita H, Comito D, et al. Asymptomatic shedding of respiratory virus among an ambulatory population across Seasons. mSphere 2018;3(4). 002499-18.
7. Rhedin S, Lindstrand A, Rotzén-Östlund M, et al. Clinical utility of PCR for common viruses in acute respiratory illness. Pediatrics 2014;133(3):e538–45.
8. Hanson KE, Azar MM, Banerjee R, et al. Molecular testing for acute respiratory tract infections: clinical and diagnostic recommendations from the IDSA's diagnostics committee. Clin Infect Dis 2020;71(10):2744–51.
9. Evans SE, Jennerich AL, Azar MM, et al. Nucleic acid-based testing for Noninfluenza viral pathogens in adults with suspected community-acquired pneumonia. An Official American Thoracic Society clinical practice guideline. Am J Respir Crit Care Med 2021;203(9):1070–87.
10. Shengchen D, Gu X, Fan G, et al. Evaluation of a molecular point-of-care testing for viral and atypical pathogens on intravenous antibiotic duration in hospitalized adults with lower respiratory tract infection: a randomized clinical trial. Clin Microbiol Infect 2019;25(11):1415–21.
11. Echavarría M, Marcone DN, Querci M, et al. Clinical impact of rapid molecular detection of respiratory pathogens in patients with acute respiratory infection. J Clin Virol 2018;108:90–5.
12. Brittain-Long R, Westin J, Olofsson S, et al. Access to a polymerase chain reaction assay method targeting 13 respiratory viruses can reduce antibiotics: a randomised, controlled trial. BMC Med 2011;9:44.
13. Brendish NJ, Malachira AK, Armstrong L, et al. Routine molecular point-of-care testing for respiratory viruses in adults presenting to hospital with acute respiratory illness (ResPOC): a pragmatic, open-label, randomised controlled trial. Lancet Respir Med 2017;5(5):401–11.
14. Baghdadi JD, O'Hara LM, Johnson JK, et al. Diagnostic stewardship to support optimal use of multiplex molecular respiratory panels: a survey from the Society for Healthcare Epidemiology of America Research Network. Infect Control Hosp Epidemiol 2023;1–6. https://doi.org/10.1017/ice.2023.72.
15. Keske Ş, Ergönül Ö, Tutucu F, et al. The rapid diagnosis of viral respiratory tract infections and its impact on antimicrobial stewardship programs. Eur J Clin Microbiol Infect Dis 2018;37(4):779–83.

16. Lowe CF, Payne M, Puddicombe D, et al. Antimicrobial stewardship for hospitalized patients with viral respiratory tract infections. Am J Infect Control 2017;45(8):872–5.
17. Srinivas P, Rivard KR, Pallotta AM, et al. Implementation of a stewardship Initiative on respiratory viral PCR-based antibiotic Deescalation. Pharmacotherapy 2019;39(6):709–17.
18. Abbas S, Bernard S, Lee KB, et al. Rapid respiratory panel testing: impact of active antimicrobial stewardship. Am J Infect Control 2019;47(2):224–5.
19. Friedman JN, Rieder MJ, Walton JM. Bronchiolitis: recommendations for diagnosis, monitoring and management of children one to 24 months of age. Paediatr Child Health 2014;19(9):485–98.
20. Weiss ZF, Cunha CB, Chambers AB, et al. Opportunities Revealed for antimicrobial stewardship and clinical practice with implementation of a rapid respiratory multiplex assay. J Clin Microbiol 2019;57(10). 008611-19.
21. Chen JHK, Lam HY, Yip CCY, et al. Clinical evaluation of the new high-Throughput Luminex NxTAG respiratory pathogen panel assay for multiplex respiratory pathogen detection. J Clin Microbiol 2016;54(7):1820–5.
22. Babady NE, England MR, Jurcic Smith KL, et al. Multicenter evaluation of the ePlex respiratory pathogen panel for the detection of viral and bacterial respiratory tract pathogens in nasopharyngeal swabs. J Clin Microbiol 2018;56(2). 016588-17.
23. Song E, Wang H, Salamon D, et al. Performance characteristics of FilmArray respiratory panel v1.7 for detection of adenovirus in a Large cohort of pediatric nasopharyngeal samples: one test may not Fit all. J Clin Microbiol 2016;54(6):1479–86.
24. Popowitch EB, O'Neill SS, Miller MB. Comparison of the Biofire FilmArray RP, Genmark eSensor RVP, Luminex xTAG RVPv1, and Luminex xTAG RVP fast multiplex assays for detection of respiratory viruses. J Clin Microbiol 2013;51(5):1528–33.
25. Leber AL, Everhart K, Daly JA, et al. Multicenter evaluation of BioFire FilmArray respiratory panel 2 for detection of viruses and bacteria in nasopharyngeal swab samples. J Clin Microbiol 2018;56(6). 019455-17.
26. Leal SM Jr, Totten AH, Xiao L, et al. Evaluation of commercial molecular diagnostic methods for detection and Determination of Macrolide resistance in Mycoplasma pneumoniae. J Clin Microbiol 2020;58(6). 002422-20.
27. Räty R, Rönkkö E, Kleemola M. Sample type is crucial to the diagnosis of Mycoplasma pneumoniae pneumonia by PCR. J Med Microbiol 2005;54(Pt 3):287–91.
28. Boman J, Allard A, Persson K, et al. Rapid diagnosis of respiratory Chlamydia pneumoniae infection by nested touchdown polymerase chain reaction compared with culture and antigen detection by EIA. J Infect Dis 1997;175(6):1523–6.
29. Den Boer JW, Yzerman EP. Diagnosis of Legionella infection in Legionnaires' disease. Eur J Clin Microbiol Infect Dis 2004;23(12):871–8.
30. Tizolova A, Guiso N, Guillot S. Insertion sequences shared by Bordetella species and implications for the biological diagnosis of pertussis syndrome. Eur J Clin Microbiol Infect Dis 2013;32(1):89–96.
31. Jerris RC, Williams SR, MacDonald HJ, et al. Testing implications of varying targets for Bordetella pertussis: comparison of the FilmArray Respiratory Panel and the Focus B. pertussis PCR assay. J Clin Pathol 2015;68(5):394–6.

32. van Asten SAV, Boers SA, de Groot JDF, et al. Evaluation of the Genmark ePlex® and QIAstat-Dx® respiratory pathogen panels in detecting bacterial targets in lower respiratory tract specimens. BMC Microbiol 2021;21(1):236.
33. Jarrett J, Uhteg K, Forman MS, et al. Clinical performance of the GenMark Dx ePlex respiratory pathogen panels for upper and lower respiratory tract infections. J Clin Virol 2021;135:104737.
34. Ruggiero P, McMillen T, Tang YW, et al. Evaluation of the BioFire FilmArray respiratory panel and the GenMark eSensor respiratory viral panel on lower respiratory tract specimens. J Clin Microbiol 2014;52(1):288–90.
35. Moradi T, Bennett N, Shemanski S, et al. Use of procalcitonin and a respiratory polymerase chain reaction panel to reduce antibiotic Use via an electronic medical record alert. Clin Infect Dis 2020;71(7):1684–9.
36. Branche AR, Walsh EE, Vargas R, et al. Serum procalcitonin Measurement and viral testing to guide antibiotic Use for respiratory infections in hospitalized adults: a randomized controlled trial. J Infect Dis 2015;212(11):1692–700.
37. Velly L, Cancella de Abreu M, Boutolleau D, et al. Point-of-care multiplex molecular diagnosis coupled with procalcitonin-guided algorithm for antibiotic stewardship in lower respiratory tract infection: a randomized controlled trial. Clin Microbiol Infect 2023. https://doi.org/10.1016/j.cmi.2023.07.031. S1198-743X(23)00359-2.
38. Serigstad S, Markussen D, Grewal HMS, et al. Rapid syndromic PCR testing in patients with respiratory tract infections reduces time to results and improves microbial yield. Sci Rep 2022;12(1):326.
39. Gilbert DN, Leggett JE, Wang L, et al. Enhanced detection of community-acquired pneumonia pathogens with the BioFire® pneumonia FilmArray® panel. Diagn Microbiol Infect Dis 2021;99(3):115246.
40. Darie AM, Khanna N, Jahn K, et al. Fast multiplex bacterial PCR of bronchoalveolar lavage for antibiotic stewardship in hospitalised patients with pneumonia at risk of Gram-negative bacterial infection (Flagship II): a multicentre, randomised controlled trial. Lancet Respir Med 2022;10(9):877–87.
41. Miller MM, Van Schooneveld TC, Stohs EJ, et al. Implementation of a rapid multiplex polymerase chain reaction pneumonia panel and subsequent antibiotic de-escalation. Open Forum Infect Dis 2023;10(8):ofad382.
42. Hughes S, Troise O, Donaldson H, et al. Bacterial and fungal coinfection among hospitalized patients with COVID-19: a retrospective cohort study in a UK secondary-care setting. Clin Microbiol Infect 2020;26(10):1395–9.
43. Gastli N, Loubinoux J, Daragon M, et al. Multicentric evaluation of BioFire FilmArray Pneumonia Panel for rapid bacteriological documentation of pneumonia. Clin Microbiol Infect 2021;27(9):1308–14.
44. Klein M, Bacher J, Barth S, et al. Multicenter evaluation of the Unyvero platform for testing bronchoalveolar lavage fluid. J Clin Microbiol 2021;59(3). 024977-20.
45. Alanio A, Hauser PM, Lagrou K, et al. ECIL guidelines for the diagnosis of Pneumocystis jirovecii pneumonia in patients with haematological malignancies and stem cell transplant recipients. J Antimicrob Chemother 2016;71(9):2386–96.
46. Zak P, Vejrazkova E, Zavrelova A, et al. BAL fluid analysis in the identification of infectious agents in patients with hematological malignancies and pulmonary infiltrates. Folia Microbiol (Praha) 2020;65(1):109–20.
47. Mühlethaler K, Bögli-Stuber K, Wasmer S, et al. Quantitative PCR to diagnose Pneumocystis pneumonia in immunocompromised non-HIV patients. Eur Respir J 2012;39(4):971–8.
48. Murphy CN, Fowler R, Balada-Llasat JM, et al. Multicenter evaluation of the BioFire FilmArray pneumonia/pneumonia plus panel for detection and quantification

of agents of lower respiratory tract infection. J Clin Microbiol 2020;58(7). e00128-20.

49. Rice S. Identifying respiratory pathogens: pneumonia panel studied against standard of care. Northfield (IL): College of American Pathologists Today Online; 2020.
50. Rand KH, Beal SG, Cherabuddi K, et al. Relationship of multiplex molecular pneumonia panel results with hospital outcomes and clinical variables. Open Forum Infect Dis 2021;8(8):ofab368.
51. Simner PJ, Dien Bard J, Doern C, et al. Reporting of antimicrobial resistance from blood cultures, an Antibacterial resistance leadership group survey summary: resistance marker reporting practices from positive blood cultures. Clin Infect Dis 2023;76(9):1550–8.
52. Yee R, Dien Bard J, Simner PJ. The genotype-to-Phenotype Dilemma: How should laboratories approach discordant susceptibility results? J Clin Microbiol 2021;59(6). 001388-20.
53. Services CfMaM. MolDX: Molecular Syndromic Panels for Infectious Disease Pathogen Identification Testing. 2022. Available at: https://www.cms.gov/medicare-coverage-database/view/lcd.aspx?lcdid=39044&ver=3.
54. Qavi AJ, McMullen A, Burnham CD, et al. Repeat molecular testing for respiratory pathogens: diagnostic gain or Diminishing Returns? J Appl Lab Med 2020;5(5): 897–907.
55. Azadeh N, Sakata KK, Brighton AM, et al. FilmArray respiratory panel assay: comparison of nasopharyngeal swabs and bronchoalveolar lavage samples. J Clin Microbiol 2015;53(12):3784–7.
56. Precit MR, He K, Mongkolrattanothai K, et al. Impact of FilmArray™ Respiratory Panel testing on the clinical management of pediatric bone marrow transplant patients. Eur J Clin Microbiol Infect Dis 2022;41(3):395–405.
57. Precit MR, Pandey U, Mongkolrattanothai K, et al. Multiplex respiratory panel repeat testing in pediatric and young adult patients infrequently offers new clinical information. J Clin Virol 2022;150-151:105168.

Diagnostic Stewardship for Next-Generation Sequencing Assays in Clinical Microbiology

An Appeal for Thoughtful Collaboration

David C. Gaston, MD, PhD[a,*], Augusto Dulanto Chiang, MD[b], Kevin Dee, MD[b], Daniel Dulek, MD[c], Ritu Banerjee, MD, PhD[d], Romney M. Humphries, PhD[a]

KEYWORDS

• Sequencing • Value • Outcomes • Best use practices • Infectious diseases

KEY POINTS

- Diagnostic stewardship is needed to increase the likelihood that a next-generation sequencing (NGS)-based assay will provide actionable results to benefit a patient.
- Collaboration between the primary care team, infectious disease consultants, clinical microbiologists, and subspecialty providers is critical for diagnostic stewardship.
- The five principles of diagnostic stewardship are to determine the best patient, syndrome, sample, timing, and test for a clinical problem. Applying these principles to the decision to pursue NGS-based testing can increase the value of this testing strategy.

INTRODUCTION

Molecular microbiology for clinical diagnostics has advanced rapidly in recent decades.[1] Polymerase chain reaction testing for individual analytes was seen as a cumbersome process when first introduced but is now readily automated with the capacity for high-volume specimen batching. The advent of highly multiplexed syndromic panels widened the analytical breadth to include the capacity to detect multiple pathogens

[a] Department of Pathology, Microbiology, and Immunology, Vanderbilt University Medical Center, 1301 Medical Center Drive TVC 4519, Nashville, TN 37232, USA; [b] Division of Infectious Diseases, Vanderbilt University Medical Center, 1211 21st Avenue South, Suite 102A, Nashville, TN 37232, USA; [c] Division of Pediatric Infectious Diseases, Vanderbilt University Medical Center, 1161 21st Avenue South, Medical Center North D7234, Nashville, TN 37232, USA; [d] Division of Pediatric Infectious Diseases, Vanderbilt University Medical Center, 1161 21st Avenue, Medical Center North D7227, Nashville, TN 37232, USA
* Corresponding author.
E-mail address: david.c.gaston@vumc.org

Clin Lab Med 44 (2024) 63–73
https://doi.org/10.1016/j.cll.2023.10.002
0272-2712/24/
labmed.theclinics.com

potentially causing a given clinical syndrome.[2] Sequencing advances follow a similar trend, transitioning from a manual process of base-calling individual nucleotides to automated massively parallel techniques evaluating multiple specimens simultaneously. Advancements in next-generation sequencing (NGS) technology enable generation of more abundant, longer, and higher quality reads, thus allowing for more accurate organism identification with lower overall costs.[3] Concurrent advancements in automation and bioinformatic analyses allow actionable result generation in a timeframe acceptable for diagnostic utility. In addition, the analytical breadth of pathogens that can be detected by NGS-based assays greatly surpasses that of contemporary multiplexed molecular approaches, and for some pathogens or instances, traditional cultures. NGS-based assays clearly have a role in the diagnosis of patients with infectious diseases. What is less clear, however, is the best utilization for NGS assays that balances the diagnostic potential with technical limitations and costs.

The topic of test implementation and use has been amply addressed in well written reviews.[4–6] However, few clinical microbiology laboratories in the United States currently possess the ability to perform in-house NGS-based testing. Barriers to implementation are decreasing, which include lower costs for sequencing equipment and reagents, increasing availability of automation for wet-laboratory steps, user-friendly bioinformatic solutions that do not require coding knowledge, and guidance from professional societies regarding assay validation, quality assurance, and quality control.[7,8] Regardless, widespread use in clinical microbiology laboratories remains limited to large academic centers or private reference laboratories. Despite this, the clinical appetite for these technologies is increasing.

The potential diagnostic impact of NGS-based assays is enticing. Case reports demonstrating resolution of elusive diagnoses can lead to a perspective that this testing can surpass, or supplant, traditional methods. Yet studies on unregulated use demonstrate low diagnostic yield and little impact on patient management, indicating a disconnect between the expected and actual performance.[9–12] This form of testing risks being overused in ways that are not beneficial for patient care. Overtesting increases the possibility of generating results that are not representative of an etiologic pathogen or simply not generating actionable results. Furthermore, poorly defined use has a real risk of undervaluing the NGS, leading to downstream consequences such as payer denial of coverage or strict hospital restrictions, which would rob such testing from patients for whom it is of value. Approaches to regulate use with the intent of improving result utility are needed. These approaches can promote testing that optimizes clinical impact while mitigating financial burdens. Such approaches can also help determine how these advancements best fit into the future of clinical microbiology in a way that is evidence-based. Best use practices are also needed to lead insurance payers and Centers for Medicare and Medicaid Services (CMS) to cover testing. Technologic developments may occur that render such regulation unnecessary, but until that point, governance with the intent of improving patient care can lead to better use of these diagnostic approaches.

CURRENTLY AVAILABLE TESTS AND THEIR LIMITATIONS

This article focuses on tests that are ordered by clinicians as part of a diagnostic workup and intended to identify pathogens directly from clinical specimens, without intermediate steps involving culture. There are two main categories of NGS-based assays that are currently available at reference laboratories in the United States: targeted amplicon sequencing and metagenomic sequencing. Targeted amplicon sequencing involves amplification of a specific region from a specimen (such as 16s ribosomal

ribosomal ribonucleic acid [rRNA] for bacteria or the internal transcribed spacer regions of fungi). NGS technologies are used to sequence the amplicons and bioinformatic processes identify the microorganism present in the initial specimen. As such, an a priori knowledge or suspicion of a specific pathogen type is needed to ensure the appropriate primers are used for amplification and the appropriate bioinformatic analyses are applied. Metagenomic sequencing attempts to sequence as many nucleic acids in a specimen as possible and determine if pathogen reads are present through bioinformatic processes. Metagenomic assays are less restricted to specific pathogen types, though their ability to detect any pathogen can be limited by the breadth of pathogens capable of being detected and whether both RNA and DNA are evaluated. Metagenomic testing casts a wide net. The net, however, may not reach deep waters.

Reference laboratories offer similar testing approaches, some with the same targets and accepted specimen sources. It is imperative to note that these assays are laboratory-developed tests and as such differ substantially in the specific methods used, many of which are proprietary. Accordingly, the analytical and clinical performance differs test-by-test and laboratory-by-laboratory. Targeted amplicon sequencing and metagenomic sequencing are categories incorporating a plurality of methods. As of yet there are no standard approaches to compare performance between assays, though these are underdevelopment.[13] The specific capabilities and limitations of a test being considered for clinical use must be understood by those caring for the patient.

Limitations broadly apply to targeted amplicon and metagenomic approaches. The most basic limitation for benchwork is that ample pathogen nucleic acids must be present in a specimen to permit detection, even for metagenomic approaches, which are often viewed as being far more sensitive. This is represented by the analytical sensitivity (limit of detection) of an assay and is a function of extraction techniques, assay targets, and the abundance of interfering host nucleic acids. If ordering targeted amplicon sequencing, the pathogen in question must be detectable by the amplification method (a fungal process will not be detected by an assay using the bacterial 16s ribosomal RNA gene as an amplification target). If ordering metagenomic sequencing, the extraction method must include the nucleic acids of the pathogen (an assay only evaluating DNA cannot detect RNA viruses). Limitations for bioinformatic analyses vary based on the analysis pipelines, but a shared limitation relates to the database used for identification. Opinions differ on the use of lower quality non-curated databases versus higher quality, less extensive curated databases.[14,15] Regardless, the performance of a bioinformatic approach depends on the presence of pathogen reads in the reference database. In addition, a general limitation for both approaches is the ability to detect nonpathogenic organisms that could be interpreted as etiologic agents of disease. Often, there are no corroborating data to support these organisms are etiologic, leading to substantial diagnostic uncertainty, particularly for immunocompromised patients. Furthermore, potentially contaminating nucleic acids can be introduced at any step of the bench process from specimen acquisition to library preparation; these may also be present in the reagents used for assays. The effects of detecting nucleic acids that are not a component of the initial specimen can be mitigated by appropriate negative controls. Even so, these assays risk detecting nucleic acids present in a testing laboratory (Labome), reagents used for testing (kitome), and other exogenous nucleic acids.[16] Finally, some reference laboratories lack clinical consulting services to help elucidate technical limitations, rendering analytical interpretation difficult. Though fundamental, these limitations can be overlooked by well-meaning providers who are unaware of the technical aspects of the testing methods, underscoring the value of both strict quality assurance programs for the laboratory and of close collaboration between laboratory and clinical care teams for interpretation of results.

Cost is a major current limitation to implementation and use. A single metagenomic test may cost approximately 2000 dollars. Although this cost pales in comparison to the cost of a single day in an intensive care unit, unmitigated use drives up cost. Further, these tests are not covered by payers for outpatients, potentially placing a large financial burden directly on a patient when not ordered in the context of an inpatient admission. If results are not actionable, patients, and payers receive no benefit for the high cost, resulting in poor value.

DISCUSSION

Diagnostic Stewardship

Diagnostic stewardship is a way to enhance assay utilization with the goal of improving patient outcomes.[17,18] The process serves as a counterbalance to well-intentioned but misdirected use. It is a critical component for the best use of current NGS-based assays because the process is not prescriptive. The best approach will vary with each patient, each presentation, and each clinical problem. This process tailors testing paradigms to an individual patient.

The process of diagnostic stewardship begins with the decision to pursue a certain testing approach and ends with result interpretation and subsequent actions. Fundamental to determining if an NGS-based assay is, or is not, the best approach is a clinical hypothesis and a robust differential diagnosis. This is the key to stewardship as it aligns the testing approach with the clinical problem. A clinical hypothesis ideally focuses on a particular pathogen that cannot (or is unlikely to) be detected by other conventional testing approaches. Alternatively, a hypothesis may be for a group of pathogens leading to a clinical syndrome, pathogens which also would not be (or have not yet been) detectable by other conventional approaches. The guidance provided by a clinical hypothesis allows the determination that a given test, with the understood limitations, has a high likelihood of detecting the suspected pathogens. If not, stewardship principles argue against pursuing that method of testing. The preferred approach carries the highest probability of identifying and characterizing an etiologic pathogen from a certain specimen taken at a particular time during an infectious syndrome. In cases where NGS-based assays are determined likely to be beneficial and ordered, the stewardship process next involves result interpretation. This step in the process evaluates the results in context of the test limitations to ensure that a valid clinical decision is made. This step may be difficult when testing is performed by a reference laboratory where the clinical team is not familiar with the test nuances or, conversely, in the absence of clinical data on the patient. Finally, the process involves continual quality improvement such that decisions made for prior patients are systematically evaluated to inform subsequent decisions.

Collaboration is essential for this process.[17] Collaboration is needed between the clinical team overseeing care, infectious disease colleagues, clinical microbiologists, and disease-specific subspecialty providers, as well as the reference laboratory medical directors and technical specialists, if testing is not performed in house. Each individual brings a differing and valuable perspective. The primary team understands the patient presentation in a wholistic manner, whereas infectious disease and subspecialty consultants are able to craft differential diagnoses to guide testing. Clinical microbiologists have an in-depth understanding of assay performance and limitations to ensure the test choice can adequately match the clinical hypothesis. All members bring similarly unique insights to the interpretation of results. Accordingly, the process of stewardship does not rest on any one individual or care team. It is a collaborative effort toward a common goal of achieving the best testing and care for a patient.

Principles of Diagnostic Stewardship

The five principles of diagnostic stewardship are to determine the best patient, the best syndrome, the best sample, the best timing, and the best test for a particular clinical problem. These principles apply for any laboratory test but are particularly apt for NGS-based assays given the overall lack of evidence-based guidance. These principles are paired with the collaborative decision to pursue testing and can be used as a guide for discussions when interpreting results. Of note, this approach assumes conventional testing approaches (culture, molecular testing, serology) have been pursued and are unrevealing or would require a lengthy turnaround time incompatible with the clinical acuity. An additional assumption is that NGS-based assays complement, not replace, conventional strategies. Although these tests are often used as a "test of last resort," good diagnostic stewardship will generate data to reveal instances where NGS may be a tool that is reached for sooner in the diagnostic journey.

Patient

The principle of the best patient for NGS-based assays relates to the medical history and predispositions for a given patient or patient population. Different populations may be benefited in different ways by the NGS-based assay type. Generally, patients who are significantly immunocompromised are deemed the most likely to benefit from testing with metagenomic assays, although these populations can also be the most complex to interpret spurious results. This preference relates to the broader array of infections to which immunocompromised patients are susceptible and the lack of robust testing approaches for certain syndromes (specifically invasive fungal infections). These are patients with solid organ transplants, hematologic stem-cell transplants, malignancies undergoing myeloablative chemotherapy, and those with primary immunodeficiencies. Patients with normally functioning immune systems can also be candidates for testing with metagenomic assays, though syndromes involving culture-negative infections in sterile sites for which serology or other molecular testing is unavailable lend to testing more than others. Targeted amplicon NGS testing is not necessarily indicated for one patient population over another, as testing is mostly performed on specimens obtained from invasive procedures. The syndrome and specimen type are stronger drivers of selecting this test type rather than underlying patient characteristics. An additional consideration is hospital admission. At present, these testing approaches are best reserved for inpatients to reserve these approaches for patients with the most severe syndromes.

Syndrome

Certain NGS-based tests are paired to specific syndromes, such as metagenomic testing on cerebrospinal fluid for patients with meningitis or encephalitis that is not attributed to an etiologic pathogen by conventional testing.[19] Others, including plasma metagenomic testing and targeted amplicon testing on various specimens, are not specifically linked to given infectious syndromes. Studies on these assays have demonstrated certain syndromes that are more likely to yield actionable results. These include neutropenic fever,[20] invasive fungal infection in patients status-post hematologic stem cell transplant,[21,22] and culture-negative syndromes, including culture negative endocarditis[23–25] or prosthetic joint infections.[26,27] Other culture negative syndromes with lower clinical severity or sequelae, such as urinary tract infections, do not fit best use guidelines for NGS-based testing. In these syndromes, the balance between obtaining an etiologic diagnosis is not offset by the potential for detecting microbiome constituents.[28] Additional syndromes may be well suited for testing with NGS-based diagnostics, but ongoing research is needed for further definition. Collaborative discussions among care teams participating in diagnostic stewardship decisions can help determine if a clinical syndrome lacking data would be appropriate for testing.

Specimen

The selection of a specimen to submit for NGS-based testing is a critical component of diagnostic stewardship. The specimen submitted needs a high probability of containing pathogen nucleic acids and a low probability of containing exogenous contaminating genetic material. For metagenomic assays, this is an aseptically collected specimen from as close to the site of infection as possible. Metagenomic testing is limited to specimen types accepted by testing laboratories, and this may not include the site of infection. Plasma metagenomic testing for cell-free DNA is capable of detecting pathogen DNA from various sites of infection. However, plasma metagenomic testing may not be the optimal choice for many syndromes with compartmentalized disease, if the site of infection is accessible.[29] Targeted amplicon sequencing for specific pathogen types is available for a larger variety of specimen sources.

If NGS-based testing is pursued, the diagnostic stewardship process must also consider specimen fidelity. Fresh frozen specimens have a higher probability of yielding a result than formalin-fixed paraffin-embedded (FFPE) specimens due to the damage to nucleic acids occurring in fixation.[30] The process of paraffin embedding is not sterile, and targeted amplicon testing performed on FFPE specimens' risks detecting environmental organisms that are not part of the specimen itself. Removing portions of an FFPE block exposed to the environment and testing from deeper sections can help prevent this, but identifying environmental organisms and potentially attributing them causality in the disease process remain a risk. A method to avoid this, and to increase the probability of obtaining actionable results, is screening the specimen for microscopic or histopathologic evidence of a pathogen before testing.[31] A best use practice for targeted amplicon sequencing or metagenomic sequencing is using the assays for pathogens that are visible in primary specimens but were not detected by conventional techniques. Visualizing pathogens by gram stain or fungal stain is a good indicator that an adequate amount of nucleic acid will be present in the specimen for detection by NGS-based assays.

Timing

The timing of specimen acquisition is ideally optimized for the syndrome being assessed. Timing is also important for potentially avoiding unnecessary interventions if testing reveals a diagnosis.[32] The optimal timing for collection is theoretically when the highest concentration of pathogen nucleic acid is present. This may not be known for a clinical syndrome, and as such it is generally assumed that the highest burden is present early in infection or when a patient is most ill. Specimen collection in this disease phase may have a higher probability of yielding actionable results, but may also be when conventional testing is ongoing. Accordingly, a practical approach is to freeze a specimen for later testing. Saving specimens has the benefit of allowing conventional testing to reveal the pathogen in a more cost-effective manner. Awaiting conventional testing may also provide characterization by culture, molecular-based techniques, or serology for which performance characteristics are more widely understood. However, freezing a specimen for later testing may not occur. If the collaborative diagnostic stewardship process determines an NGS-based assay is best for care,

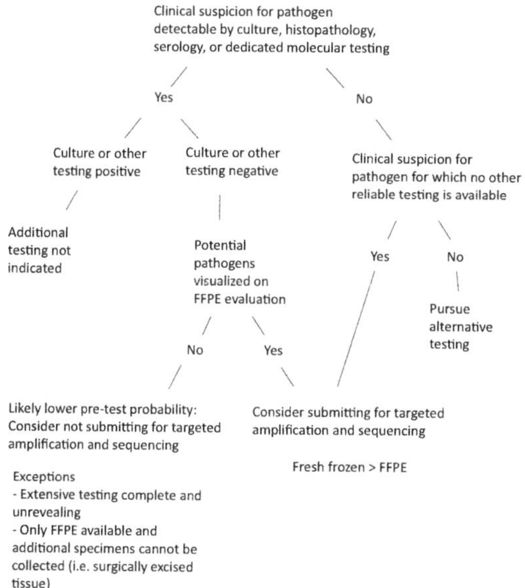

Fig. 1. Algorithm for targeted amplicon sequencing from clinical specimens.

a specimen obtained later in the course of disease may be the only option. Interpreting results in the context of when the specimen was obtained and how that can impact results is an important part of this process. Studies defining when it is best to submit a specimen for testing in various clinical syndromes are needed.

Test

Finally, determining the best test to order, based on the considerations described above, is the practical outcome of diagnostic stewardship. Conventional testing approaches may be deemed sufficient. Ensuring that the appropriate non-NGS-based testing for the patient's syndrome has been considered is a key component of the NGS diagnostic stewardship role. The use of NGS tests as a "just in case" approach following extensive, unrevealing, traditional testing should be avoided. A collaborative decision may be reached that an NGS-based test would be beneficial to care for the patient. The clinical syndrome, available specimens, and timing of disease are considered together to determine if metagenomic testing or a targeted amplicon assay would be the most likely to yield an actionable result. The proposed approaches to these decisions are outlined in **Figs. 1** and **2** and **Box 1**. Once results are available, meeting with all members engaged in the diagnostic stewardship process ensures results

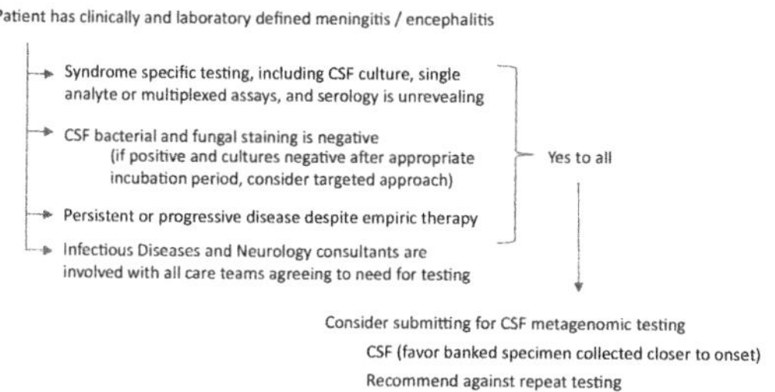

Fig. 2. The proposed criteria for cerebrospinal fluid (CSF) metagenomic testing.

Box 1
Proposed criteria for plasma metagenomic testing

Patient and syndrome are consistent with potential benefit from plasma metagenomic testing

Primary requirements (all required)

- Syndrome-specific testing, including culture, is non-diagnostic.
- Infectious diseases, microbiology, and other subspecialty consultants are involved with all care teams agreeing to need for testing.
- Plasma metagenomic testing has not been performed for the same clinical presentation.
- Intended use is not to rule out infection, as a test of cure, or as confirmatory testing after positive conventional testing.

Secondary requirements (at least two required)

- Patient is severely immunocompromised
- Clinical suspicion for invasive fungal infection
- Contraindication for obtaining tissue from site of infection for culture or targeted testing
- Patient is currently admitted
- Rapidly progressive critical illness

are effectively communicated and appropriately understood. Thereafter, a quality program that evaluates the tests ordered, utility of results, and benefit to patients can help determine how to best manage ongoing testing requests.

SUMMARY

Relatively little data currently exist on the use and benefit of NGS-based assays for infectious disease diagnostics. Additional research is needed to further define the best patients, syndromes, samples, timing, and tests for the best diagnostic approaches. A pressing need in the field is standardization of outcome measures that enable comparisons between studies using different NGS assays. A method of incorporating the principles of diagnostic stewardship into a cohesive concept is to assess an approach with the concept of value. A test that generates highly useful results that are of high quality at a relatively low cost would be an approach with great value. These variables are impacted and can be optimized by applying the diagnostic stewardship principles. Perhaps more fundamental is the need for consensus definitions that can be broadly applied in implementation studies evaluating these diagnostic approaches. It is unlikely that a single approach will be used as NGS technologies are incorporated more widely into clinical microbiology laboratories. Standardizing outcome measures that assess value, rather than standardizing technical approaches, can help evaluate differing NGS-based assays and uses.

Until best uses of NGS-based testing are defined, diagnostic stewardship practiced with a collaborative care team can determine when an NGS-based assay may best benefit a specific patient. Following diagnostic stewardship principles does not attempt to restrict testing but rather to enhance the likelihood of generating an actionable result. The process is founded in a thoughtful approach to patient care that supports the decision to pursue NGS-based testing with a clinical hypothesis and differential diagnosis. This process can help to counteract the current expense of testing and the low likelihood of generating actionable results without regulation. Stated simply, diagnostic stewardship increases the value of NGS-based testing and will benefit patient care.

CLINICS CARE POINTS

- The best use of next-generation sequencing (NGS)-based assays involves thoughtfully generating a clinical hypothesis and differential diagnosis rather than taking a "test of last resort" or hypothesis-free approach.

- NGS-based assays are currently best suited to complement, not replace, conventional microbiology testing (culture, molecular methods, and serology).
- Collaborative diagnostic stewardship teams can increase the value of testing approaches, helping to determine if and when NGS-based assays would benefit a specific patient.

DISCLOSURE

D.C. Gaston has research support from Illumina, United States and IDbyDNA, consulting for bioMerieux and DiaSorin. A.D. Chiang has no disclosures. K. Dee has no disclosures. D. Dulek has research support from Eurofins/Viracor and from NIH. R. Banerjee has research support from bioMérieux, NIH, and CDC, United States. R.M. Humphries has NGD advisory board, Advisor for Karius (unrelated to this work).

REFERENCES

1. Schmitz JE, Stratton CW, Persing DH, et al. Forty years of molecular diagnostics for infectious diseases. J Clin Microbiol 2022;60(10):e0244621.
2. Dien Bard J, McElvania E. Panels and syndromic testing in clinical microbiology. Clin Lab Med 2020;40(4):393–420.
3. Gu W, Miller S, Chiu CY. Clinical metagenomic next-generation sequencing for pathogen detection. Annu Rev Pathol 2019;14:319–38.
4. Filkins LM, Bryson AL, Miller SA, et al. Navigating clinical utilization of direct-from-specimen metagenomic pathogen detection: clinical applications, limitations, and testing recommendations. Clin Chem 2020;66(11):1381–95.
5. Dulanto Chiang A, Dekker JP. From the pipeline to the bedside: advances and challenges in clinical metagenomics. J Infect Dis 2020;221(Suppl 3):S331–40.
6. Chiu CY, Miller SA. Clinical metagenomics. Nat Rev Genet 2019;20(6):341–55.
7. Schlaberg R, Chiu CY, Miller S, et al. Validation of metagenomic next-generation sequencing tests for universal pathogen detection. Arch Pathol Lab Med 2017; 141(6):776–86.
8. Bharucha T, Oeser C, Balloux F, et al. STROBE-metagenomics: a STROBE extension statement to guide the reporting of metagenomics studies. Lancet Infect Dis 2020;20(10):e251–60.
9. Hogan CA, Yang S, Garner OB, et al. Clinical impact of metagenomic next-generation sequencing of plasma cell-free DNA for the diagnosis of infectious diseases: a multicenter retrospective cohort study. Clin Infect Dis 2021;72(2): 239–45.
10. Shishido AA, Noe M, Saharia K, et al. Clinical impact of a metagenomic microbial plasma cell-free DNA next-generation sequencing assay on treatment decisions: a single-center retrospective study. BMC Infect Dis 2022;22(1):372.
11. Niles DT, Wijetunge DSS, Palazzi DL, et al. Plasma metagenomic next-generation sequencing assay for identifying pathogens: a retrospective review of test utilization in a large children's hospital. J Clin Microbiol 2020;58(11). https://doi.org/10.1128/JCM.00794-20.
12. Niles DT, Lee RA, Lamb GS, et al. Plasma cell-free metagenomic next generation sequencing in the clinical setting for the diagnosis of infectious diseases: a systematic review and meta-analysis. Diagn Microbiol Infect Dis 2023;105(1): 115838.
13. Gaston DC. Clinical metagenomics for infectious diseases: progress toward operational value. J Clin Microbiol 2023;61(2):e0126722.

14. Breitwieser FP, Pertea M, Zimin AV, et al. Human contamination in bacterial genomes has created thousands of spurious proteins. Genome Res 2019;29(6): 954–60.
15. Steinegger M, Salzberg SL. Terminating contamination: large-scale search identifies more than 2,000,000 contaminated entries in GenBank. Genome Biol 2020; 21(1):115.
16. Simner PJ, Salzberg SL. The human "contaminome" and understanding infectious disease. N Engl J Med 2022;387(10):943–6.
17. Hueth KD, Prinzi AM, Timbrook TT. Diagnostic stewardship as a team sport: interdisciplinary perspectives on improved implementation of interventions and effect measurement. Antibiotics (Basel) 2022;11(2). https://doi.org/10.3390/antibiotics11020250.
18. Morjaria S, Chapin KC. Who to test, when, and for what: why diagnostic stewardship in infectious diseases matters. J Mol Diagn 2020;22(9):1109–13.
19. Wilson MR, Sample HA, Zorn KC, et al. Clinical metagenomic sequencing for diagnosis of meningitis and encephalitis. N Engl J Med 2019;380(24):2327–40.
20. Benamu E, Gajurel K, Anderson JN, et al. Plasma microbial cell-free DNA next-generation sequencing in the diagnosis and management of febrile neutropenia. Clin Infect Dis 2022;74(9):1659–68.
21. Hill JA, Dalai SC, Hong DK, et al. Liquid biopsy for invasive mold infections in hematopoietic cell transplant recipients with pneumonia through next-generation sequencing of microbial cell-free DNA in plasma. Clin Infect Dis 2020. https://doi.org/10.1093/cid/ciaa1639.
22. Armstrong AE, Rossoff J, Hollemon D, et al. Cell-free DNA next-generation sequencing successfully detects infectious pathogens in pediatric oncology and hematopoietic stem cell transplant patients at risk for invasive fungal disease. Pediatr Blood Cancer 2019;66(7):e27734.
23. Flurin L, Wolf MJ, Fisher CR, et al. Pathogen detection in infective endocarditis using targeted metagenomics on whole blood and plasma: a prospective pilot study. J Clin Microbiol 2022;60(9):e0062122.
24. Eichenberger EM, Degner N, Scott ER, et al. Microbial cell-free DNA identifies the causative pathogen in infective endocarditis and remains detectable longer than conventional blood culture in patients with prior antibiotic therapy. Clin Infect Dis 2023;76(3):e1492–500.
25. Hong HL, Flurin L, Greenwood-Quaintance KE, et al. 16S rRNA gene PCR/sequencing of heart valves for diagnosis of infective endocarditis in routine clinical practice. J Clin Microbiol 2023;61(8):e0034123.
26. Flurin L, Hemenway JJ, Fisher CR, et al. Clinical use of a 16S ribosomal RNA gene-based sanger and/or next generation sequencing assay to test preoperative synovial fluid for periprosthetic joint infection diagnosis. mBio 2022;13(6): e0132222.
27. Hong HL, Flurin L, Thoendel MJ, et al. Targeted versus shotgun metagenomic sequencing-based detection of microorganisms in sonicate fluid for periprosthetic joint infection diagnosis. Clin Infect Dis 2023;76(3):e1456–62.
28. Szlachta-McGinn A, Douglass KM, Chung UYR, et al. Molecular diagnostic methods versus conventional urine culture for diagnosis and treatment of urinary tract infection: a systematic review and meta-analysis. Eur Urol Open Sci 2022; 44:113–24.
29. Gu W, Deng X, Lee M, et al. Rapid pathogen detection by metagenomic next-generation sequencing of infected body fluids. Nat Med 2020. https://doi.org/10.1038/s41591-020-1105-z.

30. Cruz-Flores R, Lopez-Carvallo JA, Caceres-Martinez J, et al. Microbiome analysis from formalin-fixed paraffin-embedded tissues: current challenges and future perspectives. J Microbiol Methods 2022;196:106476.
31. Payne M, Azana R, Hoang LM. Review of 16S and ITS direct sequencing results for clinical specimens submitted to a reference laboratory. Can J Infect Dis Med Microbiol 2016;2016:4210129.
32. Fulton BD, Proudman DG, Sample HA, et al. Exploratory analysis of the potential for advanced diagnostic testing to reduce healthcare expenditures of patients hospitalized with meningitis or encephalitis. PLoS One 2020;15(1):e0226895.

The Report Says What?

How the Medical Microbiologist can aid in the Interpretation of Next-Generation Sequencing Results

Cristina Costales, MD[a,b,*], Jennifer Dien Bard, PhD[a,b]

KEYWORDS

- Metagenomic next-generation sequencing • Tumor board • Medical microbiology

KEY POINTS

- Novel applications of infectious next-generation sequencing (NGS) require the medical microbiologist be well versed in the methodology and limitations of assays available for clinical testing; ultimately, they hold responsibility for reporting quality and clinically actionable results.
- The emergence of clinical assays that utilize NGS heralds the need for a consistent reporting algorithm, especially around quantitation of microbes identified and their probable clinical significance.
- Communicating results of NGS testing ideally involves direct interaction of the medical microbiologist with the clinical team, such that experts on testing methodology can candidly exchange findings and concerns with patient care professionals.

INTRODUCTION

As precision medicine evolves and access to complex infectious molecular testing in the clinical environment continues to become more widely available, the medical microbiologist increasingly becomes an essential conduit for translating complicated sequencing data into actionable pathogen information for the practicing clinician.

A key aspect of the medical microbiologist's role, in addition to acting as diagnostic steward, is to ensure high quality and clinically actionable data are transmitted to the patient's provider.[1] Thus, it is imperative that medical microbiologists take an active, vigilant approach of reporting microbial molecular results, especially as the complexity

[a] Department of Pathology and Laboratory Medicine, Children's Hospital Los Angeles, Los Angeles, CA, USA; [b] Keck School of Medicine, University of Southern California, Los Angeles, CA, USA
* Corresponding author. Children's Hospital Los Angeles, 4650 Sunset Boulevard MS32, Los Angeles, CA 90027.
E-mail address: ccostales@chla.usc.edu

Clin Lab Med 44 (2024) 75–84
https://doi.org/10.1016/j.cll.2023.10.006

of molecular techniques increases. Even for those sequencing assays used by clinical teams but not developed in-house as a laboratory-developed test (LDT), medical microbiologists are obligated to have a working understanding of the methodology, opportunities for stewardship, and assay limitations. Until next-generation sequencing (NGS) testing becomes routine in the clinical laboratory, it is arguable that the scenario of sending testing to a reference laboratory would be the norm. Thus, it would behoove the microbiologist to collaborate with the rest of the clinical team as the subject matter expert when interpreting the results. Undoubtedly, clinical pressure will continue to mount for utilization of these methods across multiple medical fields. Microbiologists would do well to self-educate on the methods, and in particular, interpretation of results, lest other facets of the medical community not recognize the importance of microbiology expertise in the wake of these powerful technologies.[2]

Although extensive guidance documents for testing utilization of infectious metagenomic NGS (mNGS) or microbial whole-genome sequencing (WGS) are not yet available,[3] microbiologists should work with their infectious disease colleagues to develop testing algorithms to identify the patients that would most benefit from these still expensive tests. Further, testing algorithms should also include defined criteria for interpretation and reporting of organisms, resistance genes, pathogenicity markers, and even host-response markers as the technology progresses.[4] When clinically applicable and logistically practical, the laboratory analyses and reporting scheme should differentiate between incidental and clinically relevant findings, and reports results in a way that supports appropriate therapeutic decision-making as per regulatory criteria.[5] In this article, we will discuss the important factors to consider for developing laboratory reporting criteria and how to effectively translate the results of infectious NGS testing.

APPLICATIONS OF NEXT-GENERATION SEQUENCING IN CLINICAL MICROBIOLOGY

As discussed in the prior articles in this issue, the applications of NGS in the clinical microbiology laboratory continue to expand, as the technology becomes more accessible and less cost and time prohibitive. Whether offered as an LDT in-house, LDT at a reference laboratory, or commercially available, several applications of this method are available.

Targeted Next-Generation Sequencing

For more than 2 decades, first-generation Sanger sequencing methods have been used for pathogen identifications in the clinical laboratory.[6] For unidentified bacterial, mycobacterial, or fungal species from isolates or primary specimens, assays are designed to target and amplify the conserved and variable regions of ribosomal RNA, and other similar conserved genes to allow for species level identification. The Clinical and Laboratory Standards Institute has provided detailed consensus guidance for reporting criteria for these targeted assays.[7] These standards include quality metrics for assigning an isolated pathogen to species or genus level, with caveats noted for the resolution of particular organisms and the appropriate ribosomal region targets.[7] Many of these criteria can be applied to pathogen identification by next-generation targeted sequencing assays because most use the same selection (via polymerase chain reaction [PCR] amplification/deep amplicon sequencing) or enrichment (via probe hybridization) of bacterial and fungal targets. Although some assays have added RNA extraction and probe enrichment steps to include viral targets, bacterial and fungal results details can be at least partially adopted from these well-established parameters.[8]

Unbiased or Shotgun Metagenomic Next-Generation Sequencing

Although mNGS allows for an unbiased approach to pathogen detection, extensive experience with targeted molecular testing in the clinical laboratory highlights the fact that not all pathogen detection correlates with clinical infection or disease. Further, the complex methods that allow for unbiased mNGS detection imbue a potential for error that must be well understood by the medical microbiologist responsible for reporting these results.[9]

Although general guidelines for reporting results of microbial mNGS research have been suggested by the STROBE-metagenomics group,[10] similar parameters may guide clinical reporting, as well as factors to consider in the validation of an mNGS assay.[11] Many of these NGS parameters relate to reducing potential sources of bias, most of which would be addressed and minimized through the standardization of the methodology required for clinical validation.[9,11] With unbiased sequencing, additional interfering nucleic acids from the host or nonpathogens add complexity to interpretation that must be addressed when developing the bioinformatics pipeline.[4] The microbiologist would also consider the impact that interfering nucleic acids may have on the overall sensitivity when communicating the interpretation of the results with the other clinical teams.

Antimicrobial Susceptibility Testing

Including antimicrobial resistance genes in the same assays developed for pathogen detection has been proposed as the next step in infectious NGS testing, either by way of WGS of isolates or included in the metagenomic sequencing pipeline.[12–16] Although the same issues originate in predicting phenotypic susceptibility of an organism using only genomic data as with targeted antimicrobial resistance gene PCR assays,[17] the promise of a one-stop shop for pathogen identification, susceptibility profile, and pathogenicity is intriguing.[6] This additional actionable data of the pathogenicity/therapeutic options adds value to a testing scheme that, at least currently, cost outweighs the value returned as compared with standard microbiology methods.[18]

An additional factor preventing application of NGS for microbial susceptibility in the clinical laboratory, relates to the lack of correlation between genotypic resistance profiles and clinically validated phenotypic data.[6] Although significant progress has been made in this regard, with such databanks as the Comprehensive Antibiotic Resistance Database,[19] there is still a vast need for clinical outcome data for genomic identified resistance markers. Thus, the requirement for phenotypic AST will likely remain, even with evolution and further implementation of genotypic testing.[6,17]

Microbiome Profiling and Resistome Applications

Although not yet available as an assay in clinical laboratories, mNGS methods are rapidly paving the way for reporting an individual patient's microbiome environment and resistome profile, the holy grail of precision medicine. By avoiding amplification, third-generation sequencing methods (ie, Nanopore) can produce results that accurately reflect the diversity and proportions of microbial populations in a given sample and can do so in a rapid manner for truly actionable influence on the patient.[20–23] There has been much interest in the exploration of urinary microbiome and vaginal microbiome testing to aid in the diagnosis of urinary tract and gynecologic infections, respectively.[24] There are some commercial laboratories that currently offer these services but the clinical relevance remains to be determined and is currently not considered acceptable diagnostic practice.[25,26]

Respiratory microbiome profiling is another area of active interest because standard microbiology culture methods may fail to elucidate the complex microbial interactions in those patients with chronic lung diseases.[22] Although still in early stages of development as clinical tests, the groups are moving toward this unbiased approach for faster and more sensitive pathogen detection.[21] Again the caveat here, similar to what laboratories have experienced with multiplex PCR for pneumonia, correlating pathogen detection with respiratory infection and true disease, will need to be shown through exhaustive clinical utility studies in a wide variety of patient populations, along with careful consideration for organism reporting.[27]

RESOLVING CONTAMINANTS IN NEXT-GENERATION SEQUENCING TESTING

Contamination with environmental microbes has been an issue in the microbiology laboratory since the emergence of the field in Pasteur's laboratory. Clinical microbiologic procedures have incrementally improved to reduce the noise from unwanted environmental and commensal organisms worked up and reported from culture. The microbiologist is familiar with the broad spectrum of common laboratory/environmental contaminants recovered through standard methods and similarly will need to become acquainted with the genomic environmental contaminants frequently detected by mNGS methods. Although viable contaminant microorganisms may persist on collection and specimen processing devices, contaminant microbial DNA and RNA is far more ubiquitous, and persists in reagents and other laboratory supplies, in addition to the microbial genetic elements within the blood, tissue, or body fluid specimen itself.[28,29] Thus, mNGS pathogen-detection methods must include relative quantitation of each identified microbe in the form of z-scores, from which clinical relevance can be interpreted either by a medical microbiologist/pathologist[30] or increasingly through machine learning algorithms.[31]

As powerfully sensitive new tools become increasingly available through molecular methods, with the same risk of contaminant recovery, laboratories must also consider how to report organisms in a systematic way to avoid overtreatment of nonpathogenic entities. As NGS assays become more complex and incorporate more elements of pathogen and host data, so too does the interpretation and need for clear, consistent reporting.

RESULT REPORTING ALGORITHMS

As per current College of American Pathologists (CAP) recommendations, for those with in-house NGS platforms responsible for final interpretation and reporting of NGS results, each laboratory must hold written algorithm for reporting infectious testing.[5] This algorithm must include a system to classify the clinical significance of any identified organisms. If reporting on antimicrobial resistance markers or other host-response markers, these genes must also be quantified by clinical relevance.[15,32] Key parameters of this algorithm include distinction between microbial nucleic acid from the environment, clinically insignificant normal flora microbial organisms, and clinically relevant likely pathogens.[1,9] These reports would benefit from the inclusion of clinical consultation note from the microbiologist with interpretative guidance of molecular findings, particularly with the detection of microbial flora with low likelihood of disease association.

One pertinent example in which microbiologist interpretation could be critical to avoid misdiagnosis and overuse of antibiotics is that of *Enterococcus cecorum* as detected from plasma cell-free mNGS. This organism is a known livestock commensal and poultry pathogen with only very rare human infections reported usually with close zoonotic contact,[33] yet it has also been noted to be detected via mNGS in low quantity in association with the drug defibrotide. Defibrotide is used to prevent hepatic veno-occlusive disease in hematopoietic cell transplant (HCT) patients and is derived from porcine intestinal DNA.[34] The plausible explanation for the detection of *E cecorum* in a hospitalized HCT patient without exposure to animals is that genetic components of the organism are picked up by deep sequencing of the depolymerized porcine intestinal DNA. Thus, correlation and interpretation of any potential pathogen detected by mNGS methods, particularly at low levels or below the level of quantitation, should be thoroughly reviewed and reported with context for the microorganism identified.

Reliable creation of sequencing libraries from negative controls presumes a steady state of background microbial molecular elements, either in wet laboratory reagents or from the specimen type itself, which is a known fallacy.[29,30] Although groups are actively pursuing dynamic algorithms that account for these inconsistencies in a low-level microbial baseline, they are far from clinical implementation across reporting laboratories.[29]

Although molecular pathology groups, including the American College of Medical Genetics and Association for Molecular Pathology, have developed extensive guidelines for the interpretation of sequence variants in genomic NGS testing, a framework for such standardized reporting does not yet exist for the interpretation of microbial/infectious sequencing.[35] This becomes more complex for reporting WGS results with pathogenicity implications and for reporting resistance markers. In addition to using standardized language for reporting variants, these reports will have to include clinically relevant information. On the forefront of development of worldwide standard for NGS nomenclature and reporting is a global consortium, which has published specific templates for *Mycobacterium tuberculosis* WGS.[14] This template consists of a clinician-facing report with simplified interpretive criteria for patient treatment based on high-confidence drug resistance mutations identified, ideal for practitioners less familiar with NGS methods and a secondary report that details more comprehensive data-set including nuanced NGS variables for experienced user consultation.[14]

Another example of the need for standardized reporting became known during the coronavirus disease 2019 pandemic, in which multiple clinical laboratories rapidly implemented WGS for severe acute respiratory syndrome coronavirus 2. Recommended reporting criteria included listing the sequencing method, significant variants detected, and a section for clinical interpretation, including potential therapeutic impact.[36] Similar reporting templates may be applied to mNGS pathogen detection and WGS assays.

IN-HOUSE VERSUS EXTERNAL REFERENCE LABORATORY REPORTING

Laboratory-developed sequencing assays afford the clinical microbiologist opportunities to tailor bioinformatics and sequencing analyses to their hospital's specific patient population. This includes setting thresholds for reporting as well as developing customized reporting framework.[37]

When infectious NGS testing is performed externally, the medical microbiologist is still responsible, with input from clinical colleagues, for selecting a reference laboratory NGS assay that meets patient population needs and accreditation standards. The microbiologist may have oversight of what specimens are sent out from the hospital for molecular testing but in many instances may not; thus, it is imperative to become familiar with the methods and reporting parameters of molecular testing performed at affiliate reference laboratories. This is particularly important when broad range targets for sequencing or metagenomic sequencing are used because specimen quality may not be evaluated before send out.[6] When possible, the microbiologist may consider establishing a process with colleagues from reference or commercial laboratories to ensure that they receive the report before its availability in the electronic medical record. This would allow them to pursue consultation with the infectious diseases team or other relevant clinical teams to discuss the result and provide interpretative input.

TUMOR BOARD STYLE DISCUSSION OF RESULTS

Ideally, results from metagenomic sequencing will provide pathogen identification that have been screened for contaminants via validated bioinformatics algorithms[29] and assume a plausible cause for the patient's presentation. Such automated bioinformatics pipelines validated for clinical use are likely still several years in the future.[30] Until the trust in these NGS assays is established, a potential approach to result interpretation may lay in an organized discussion among health-care teams involved, including but not limited to medical microbiologists and/or molecular specialist laboratory scientists, infectious disease physicians, hospitalists, pulmonologists, and transplant care team members depending on patient characteristics and site-specific testing.[37] This is modeled from multidisciplinary oncology molecular tumor boards wherein specialists meet to plan optimized therapy in response to imaging, pathology, and, increasingly, NGS molecular results of solid or hematologic malignancies.[38] Certain patient populations that may require specialist insight including those with cystic fibrosis,[39] febrile neutropenia,[40,41] chronic meningitis,[42] and other disease areas with potential caveats to pathogen versus opportunistic microbe interpretation.

Microbiologists would ideally lead these discussions to guide the clinical interpretation of findings *directly* to the clinical teams involved in the patient's care. Direct communication with the primary teams, rather than having Infectious Diseases colleagues serve as the liaison, would be ideal to foster consultative and collaborative relationships. Several points to be addressed with each patient's sequencing results include the following:

1. Interpretation of results in the clinical context.
   Here the clinicians familiar with the patient's presentation, underlying immune status, exposure history, and infectious history are key for correlation of microbial elements identified through the NGS pipeline.
2. Discussion of sequencing reads below the established cutoff or identifications from supplementary analysis of NGS data.
   Clinical insight gained from physician specialists may bring to light potential pathogens reads below the level of the validated analysis path, which must be set at relatively conservative thresholds to maintain method specificity.[9]
3. Correlation with standard microbial methods and ancillary testing for pathogens identified by NGS.
   Opportunity for microbiologist to compare the sensitivity of standard infectious diagnostics to mNGS results and identify situations in which additional confirmatory or ancillary testing may be needed, particularly for cases with negative mNGS results despite clear evidence of infectious cause of symptoms.

For those laboratorians unable to meet physically or virtually with clinical colleagues, the report generated should be of sufficient detail, including literature references and detailed description of quantitation methodology, such that clinicians may make informed decisions.

Host response profile will be discussed in the next article but because these methods become more widely available or included into mNGS assays, incorporating and testing the clinical utility of these factors may dramatically affect the microbial identification interpretation.[31,43]

TRACKING CLINICAL IMPACT

For academic centers with clinical mNGS testing systems in use, it is imperative that the medical microbiologist monitor how reported sequencing data are used by the clinical team. This will help to delineate testing algorithms for disease parameters and specimen types to include or exclude from metagenomic testing based on the relevance of the data for that patient. For instance, when metagenomic testing is applied to disease states with altered microflora environments such as cystic fibrosis, feedback to the clinical laboratory on how reported organism data (longitudinal quantitation, resistome profile) is used to guide treatment, may in turn inform the threshold for reporting certain organisms.[39] Some specimen types such as respiratory collections may require alternate thresholds for reporting, similar to how culture workup is performed.

For plasma cell-free mNGS testing, which has been commercially available for several years, the clinical utility ranges from 7% and 14% across various institutions[44,45] and with higher clinical impact noted in immunocompromised patient populations.[41,46,47] These published studies demonstrate the need for continued data acquisition in assessing the real-time clinical impact of cell-free mNGS, in particular how the method compares to standard microbiology results and the decision tree for change in therapy based on NGS results.

REIMBURSEMENT WOES

Although the numerous case reports in which mNGS recognized an otherwise unidentifiable pathogen argue that any life-saving intervention is worth the expense, any clinical laboratorian with fiscal responsibilities will need additional evidence of clinical impact and improved yield over standard testing methods before adopting NGS as a routine test. For instance, in comparing mNGS to commercial multiplex PCR panels, we may see some improved sensitivity with the mNGS method especially (and obviously) with off-panel targets[48]; however, until reimbursement for this type of testing is addressed, the use of the test will be limited to large academic institutes that are able to absorb the cost of testing. In many incidences, the cost burden falls onto the laboratory operation budget.

Because payers, both public and private, coverage decisions are largely based on proven clinical utility of a test,[49] additional evidence for the impact of mNGS testing on medical practice is warranted. One way that early adopters of the technology can contribute is to develop standardized reporting of microbial NGS data for clinical use and publication that allow for straightforward interpretation of results.

SUMMARY

As we have seen with other technologies adopted in the clinical microbiology laboratory, from mass spectrometry to multiplex syndromic panels to rapid susceptibility interpretation, the key to integration is providing clinicians with an interpretable result that leads to improved clinical actionability.[30] Herein lies a critical task for the medical microbiologist: to navigate the evermore complex world of NGS testing and produce clear, standardized reporting that directly influences patient care.

REFERENCES

1. Gaston DC, Miller HB, Fissel JA, et al. Evaluation of metagenomic and targeted next-generation sequencing workflows for detection of respiratory pathogens from Bronchoalveolar Lavage fluid specimens. J Clin Microbiol 2022;60(7): e0052622.
2. Lakbar I, Singer M, Leone M. 2030:will we still need our microbiologist? Intensive Care Med 2023. https://doi.org/10.1007/s00134-023-07186-6.
3. Miller JM, Binnicker MJ, Campbell S, et al. A guide to utilization of the microbiology laboratory for diagnosis of infectious diseases: 2018 update by the infectious diseases Society of America and the American Society for microbiology. Clin Infect Dis 2018;67(6):813–6.
4. Miller S, Chiu C. The role of metagenomics and next-generation sequencing in infectious disease diagnosis. Clin Chem 2021;68(1):115–24.
5. Aziz N, Zhao Q, Bry L, et al. College of American Pathologists' laboratory standards for next-generation sequencing clinical tests. Arch Pathol Lab Med 2015;139(4):481–93.
6. Church DL, Cerutti L, Gürtler A, et al. Performance and application of 16S rRNA gene cycle sequencing for routine identification of bacteria in the clinical microbiology laboratory. Clin Microbiol Rev 2020;33(4). https://doi.org/10.1128/CMR.00053-19.
7. Interpretive Criteria for identification of bacteria and fungi by targeted DNA sequencing. In: CLSI Guideline MM18. 2nd edition. Wayne, PA: Clinical and Laboratory Standards Institute; 2018.
8. Hilt EE, Ferrieri P. Next generation and other sequencing technologies in diagnostic microbiology and infectious diseases. Genes 2022;13(9). https://doi.org/10.3390/genes13091566.
9. Schlaberg R, Chiu CY, Miller S, et al. Validation of metagenomic next-generation sequencing tests for universal pathogen detection. Arch Pathol Lab Med 2017; 141(6):776–86.
10. Bharucha T, Oeser C, Balloux F, et al. STROBE-metagenomics: a STROBE extension statement to guide the reporting of metagenomics studies. Lancet Infect Dis 2020;20(10):e251–60.
11. Miller S, Naccache SN, Samayoa E, et al. Laboratory validation of a clinical metagenomic sequencing assay for pathogen detection in cerebrospinal fluid. Genome Res 2019;29(5):831–42.
12. Ellington MJ, Ekelund O, Aarestrup FM, et al. The role of whole genome sequencing in antimicrobial susceptibility testing of bacteria: report from the EUCAST Subcommittee. Clin Microbiol Infect 2017;23(1):2–22.
13. Tamma PD, Fan Y, Bergman Y, et al. Applying rapid whole-genome sequencing to predict phenotypic antimicrobial susceptibility testing results among carbapenem-resistant Klebsiella pneumoniae clinical isolates. Antimicrob Agents Chemother 2019;63(1). https://doi.org/10.1128/AAC.01923-18.
14. Tornheim JA, Starks AM, Rodwell TC, et al. Building the framework for standardized clinical laboratory reporting of next-generation sequencing data for resistance-associated mutations in Mycobacterium tuberculosis complex. Clin Infect Dis 2019;69(9):1631–3.
15. Weinmaier T, Conzemius R, Bergman Y, et al. Validation and application of Long-read whole-genome sequencing for antimicrobial resistance gene detection and antimicrobial susceptibility testing. Antimicrob Agents Chemother 2023;67(1): e0107222.

16. Allicock OM, Guo C, Uhlemann AC, et al. BacCapSeq: a platform for diagnosis and characterization of bacterial infections. mBio 2018;9(5). https://doi.org/10.1128/mBio.02007-18.
17. Bard JD, Lee F. Why can't we just use PCR? The role of genotypic versus phenotypic testing for antimicrobial resistance testing. Clin Microbiol Newsl 2018; 40(11):87–95.
18. Miller S, Chiu C, Rodino KG, et al. Point-counterpoint: should we Be performing metagenomic next-generation sequencing for infectious disease diagnosis in the clinical laboratory? J Clin Microbiol 2020;58(3). https://doi.org/10.1128/JCM.01739-19.
19. Alcock BP, Huynh W, Chalil R, et al. Card 2023: expanded curation, support for machine learning, and resistome prediction at the Comprehensive Antibiotic Resistance Database. Nucleic Acids Res 2023;51(D1):D690–9.
20. Schmidt K, Mwaigwisya S, Crossman LC, et al. Identification of bacterial pathogens and antimicrobial resistance directly from clinical urines by nanopore-based metagenomic sequencing. J Antimicrob Chemother 2017;72(1):104–14.
21. Charalampous T, Kay GL, Richardson H, et al. Nanopore metagenomics enables rapid clinical diagnosis of bacterial lower respiratory infection. Nat Biotechnol 2019;37(7):783–92.
22. Chapman R, Jones L, D'Angelo A, et al. Nanopore-based metagenomic sequencing in respiratory tract infection: a developing diagnostic platform. Lung 2023;201(2):171–9.
23. Gu W, Deng X, Lee M, et al. Rapid pathogen detection by metagenomic next-generation sequencing of infected body fluids. Nat Med 2021;27(1):115–24.
24. Kawalec A, Zwolińska D. Emerging role of microbiome in the prevention of urinary tract infections in children. Int J Mol Sci 2022;23(2). https://doi.org/10.3390/ijms23020870.
25. Kim MJ, Lee S, Kwon MY, et al. Clinical significance of composition and functional diversity of the vaginal microbiome in recurrent vaginitis. Front Microbiol 2022;13: 851670.
26. Zhang L, Huang W, Zhang S, et al. Rapid detection of bacterial pathogens and antimicrobial resistance genes in clinical urine samples with urinary tract infection by metagenomic nanopore sequencing. Front Microbiol 2022;13:858777.
27. Edgeworth JD. Respiratory metagenomics: route to routine service. Curr Opin Infect Dis 2023;36(2):115–23.
28. Dulanto Chiang A, Dekker JP. From the pipeline to the Bedside: advances and challenges in clinical metagenomics. J Infect Dis 2020;221(Suppl 3):S331–40.
29. Du J, Zhang J, Zhang D, et al. Background filtering of clinical metagenomic sequencing with a library concentration-normalized model. Microbiol Spectr 2022;10(5):e0177922.
30. Greninger AL. The challenge of diagnostic metagenomics. Expert Rev Mol Diagn 2018;18(7):605–15.
31. Kalantar KL, Neyton L, Abdelghany M, et al. Integrated host-microbe plasma metagenomics for sepsis diagnosis in a prospective cohort of critically ill adults. Nat Microbiol 2022;7(11):1805–16.
32. Mitchell SL, Simner PJ. Next-generation sequencing in clinical microbiology: are we there yet? Clin Lab Med 2019;39(3):405–18.
33. Lundy A, Claudinon A, Tirolien JA, et al. Purpura fulminans due to. IDCases 2022; 29:e01522.

34. Richardson PG, Palomo M, Kernan NA, et al. The importance of endothelial protection: the emerging role of defibrotide in reversing endothelial injury and its sequelae. Bone Marrow Transplant 2021;56(12):2889–96.
35. Richards S, Aziz N, Bale S, et al. Standards and guidelines for the interpretation of sequence variants: a joint consensus recommendation of the American College of medical genetics and genomics and the association for molecular pathology. Genet Med 2015;17(5):405–24.
36. Greninger AL, Dien Bard J, Colgrove RC, et al. Clinical and infection prevention applications of Severe acute respiratory Syndrome coronavirus 2 genotyping: an infectious diseases Society of America/American Society for microbiology consensus review document. Clin Infect Dis 2022;74(8):1496–502.
37. Wilson MR, Sample HA, Zorn KC, et al. Clinical metagenomic sequencing for diagnosis of meningitis and encephalitis. N Engl J Med 2019;380(24):2327–40.
38. Jain NM, Schmalz L, Cann C, et al. Framework for implementing and tracking a molecular tumor board at a National cancer Institute-designated comprehensive cancer center. Oncol 2021;26(11):e1962–70.
39. Bacci G, Taccetti G, Dolce D, et al. Untargeted metagenomic investigation of the Airway microbiome of cystic fibrosis patients with moderate-Severe lung disease. Microorganisms 2020;8(7). https://doi.org/10.3390/microorganisms8071003.
40. Vijayvargiya P, Feri A, Mairey M, et al. Metagenomic shotgun sequencing of blood to identify bacteria and viruses in leukemic febrile neutropenia. PLoS One 2022; 17(6):e0269405.
41. Benamu E, Gajurel K, Anderson JN, et al. Plasma microbial cell-free DNA next-generation sequencing in the diagnosis and management of febrile neutropenia. Clin Infect Dis 2022;74(9):1659–68.
42. Wilson MR, O'Donovan BD, Gelfand JM, et al. Chronic meningitis investigated via metagenomic next-generation sequencing. JAMA Neurol 2018;75(8):947–55.
43. Cheng AP, Burnham P, Lee JR, et al. A cell-free DNA metagenomic sequencing assay that integrates the host injury response to infection. Proc Natl Acad Sci U S A 2019;116(37):18738–44.
44. Hogan CA, Yang S, Garner OB, et al. Clinical impact of metagenomic next-generation sequencing of plasma cell-free DNA for the diagnosis of infectious diseases: a multicenter retrospective cohort Study. Clin Infect Dis 2021;72(2): 239–45.
45. Lee RA, Al Dhaheri F, Pollock NR, et al. Assessment of the clinical utility of plasma metagenomic next-generation sequencing in a pediatric hospital population. J Clin Microbiol 2020;24(7). https://doi.org/10.1128/JCM.00419-20.
46. Niles DT, Lee RA, Lamb GS, et al. Plasma cell-free metagenomic next generation sequencing in the clinical setting for the diagnosis of infectious diseases: a systematic review and meta-analysis. Diagn Microbiol Infect Dis 2023;105(1): 115838.
47. Rossoff J, Chaudhury S, Soneji M, et al. Noninvasive diagnosis of infection using plasma next-generation sequencing: a Single-center experience. Open Forum Infect Dis 2019;6(8). https://doi.org/10.1093/ofid/ofz327.
48. Graf EH, Simmon KE, Tardif KD, et al. Unbiased detection of respiratory viruses by use of RNA sequencing-based metagenomics: a systematic comparison to a commercial PCR panel. J Clin Microbiol 2016;54(4):1000–7.
49. Deverka PA, Kaufman D, McGuire AL. Overcoming the reimbursement barriers for clinical sequencing. JAMA 2014;312(18):1857–8.

Is It Possible to Test for Viral Infectiousness?

The Use Case of (SARS-CoV-2)

Heba H. Mostafa, MD, PhD

KEYWORDS

• Infectiousness • Transmissibility • Cycle threshold • SARS-CoV-2 • COVID-19
• sgRNA

KEY POINTS

- Testing for infectiousness is a clinical and public health need, but a diagnostic stewardship controversy.
- Recovering infectious virus in cell culture has been considered the gold standard for testing for infectiousness.
- Various approaches, including the use of cycle threshold values and antigen testing, have been used to estimate infectiousness.
- Currently, there are no specific tests available for directly determining infectiousness.

INTRODUCTION AND DEFINITIONS

The gold standard for the diagnosis of the majority of infections with viral pathogens is primarily nucleic acid amplification. Using this sensitive approach, viral nucleic acid has been detected for an extended period after the initial diagnosis, challenging the distinction between the detection of viral nucleic acid shedding versus the detection of infectious virus.[1–7] The Coronavirus Disease 2019 (COVID-19) pandemic highlighted the significance of this challenge, as there was a continuous need to define isolation time, patients' quarantine, and treatment courses. Various approaches were used to estimate patients' infectiousness, including relative virus loads (cycle threshold [Ct] values), antigen tests, and subgenomic ribonucleic acid (sgRNA). The recovery of infectious virus in cell culture has been the strongest evidence of infectiousness; however, its utility has been limited primarily due to the high biosafety level required for virus growth and isolation. Defining the minimum infectious dose that determines virus transmissibility, along with standardizing methods of viral quantification and isolation, can help establish infectiousness cutoffs.

Johns Hopkins School of Medicine, Meyer B-121F, 600 North Wolfe Street, Baltimore, MD 21287, USA
E-mail address: Hmostaf2@jhmi.edu

Clin Lab Med 44 (2024) 85–93
https://doi.org/10.1016/j.cll.2023.10.008
labmed.theclinics.com

Infectiousness: The presence of infectious virus particles on an individual level. Infectiousness refers to the individual's ability to transmit the infection.[8]

Transmissibility: The ability of the virus to transmit from an infected individual to a contact.[8] Transmission depends on the presence of infectious virus; however, its efficiency is multifactorial and can be influenced by variables such as humidity, distance, exposure time, and preexisting immunity.

CYCLE THRESHOLD VALUES

Ct values reflect the number of cycles required for the fluorescent signal during real-time amplification to cross the threshold of the assay, and they serve, in a qualitatively developed assay, as indicators of positive versus negative target amplification. An inverse relationship between the target amount and Ct value is expected. However, for qualitative assays, accurate quantitative nucleic acid measurements based on Ct values alone cannot be provided. Multiple factors that may not have been optimized during the development of qualitative assays could impact the reliability of accurate relative quantification.[9] Most importantly is the lack of a validated calibration curve that could translate a Ct value to an accurate quantity. Ct values were extensively used during the COVID-19 pandemic to guide infection control and patients' management.[10–12] Molecular platforms with lower analytical sensitivity but faster turnaround times, such as ID NOW by Abbott, were accepted for diagnosis, based on assumptions that lower relative viral loads are associated with less likelihood of infectiousness.[13] In one study, a cutoff Ct value of greater than 30 was used for infection control and isolation decisions,[14] among other examples where Ct values, as an equivalent for relative viral loads, were used as a proxy for infectiousness.

Does the Likelihood of a Patient's Infectiousness Decrease If Severe acute respiratory syndrome coronavirus 2 (SARS-CoV-2) RNA Is Detected at High Cycle Threshold Values (ie, Lower Viral Load)?

Ct values correlated with viral RNA copies and with TCID50 (50% tissue culture infectious dose), which is an endpoint dilution assay used to measure infectious viral titer, when serial dilutions of a viral stock were used to infect Vero E6 cells.[15] A low average Ct value was the most consistent variable associated with the successful recovery of infectious virus from nasal and nasopharyngeal swabs in cell culture.[16–20] However, samples with low Ct values were not consistently associated with the recovery of infectious virus on multiple occasions, whereas samples with Ct values higher than 30 occasionally tested positive in cell culture. The interquartile range of Ct values of samples associated with positive versus negative recovery of infectious virus consistently showed marked overlap,[16,18] highlighting the limitation of defining a cutoff that could be used at an individual patient level. In addition, the recovery of infectious virus in cell culture was affected by the individuals' vaccination status, indicating that variables other than Ct values are likely to impact infectiousness. Importantly, neutralizing antibodies play a significant role in this regard.[19,20] Recovering infectious virus in relation to the course of infection and the onset of symptoms was also studied. The peak shedding of viral RNA was estimated to occur on day 4 after the onset of symptoms (which might slightly vary by viral variant[21] and community-level immune status[22]), and the recovery of infectious virus was predominantly observed during the first week of symptoms.[3,17] Based on this, according to most initial guidelines, the first 10 days of symptoms were considered potentially infectious, as well as the first 10 days after a positive test in asymptomatic people. Isolation measures were primarily recommended during this time frame.[1] However, the recovery phase has been characterized by prolonged RNA shedding, and many reports have shown the recovery of infectious virus beyond the 10-day time frame, especially in immunocompromised patients.[23–26]

Are Patients with Severe Acute Respiratory Syndrome Coronavirus 2 (SARS-CoV-2) RNA Detected at High Cycle Threshold Values Unable to Transmit Infectious Virus Particles?

Because recovering infectious virus in cell culture cannot be simply translated into transmissibility, it becomes important to understand the correlation between Ct values and viral transmission to secondary contacts. Although viral transmission can be influenced by many environmental and host factors, the viral load in the upper respiratory compartment is expected to be a significant variable. An index case with a viral load of $< 1 \times 10^6$ was associated with a slightly reduced likelihood of transmission when compared with index cases with loads $> 1 \times 10$^6 copies/mL.[27] Transmission is also affected by the course of the infection, with the majority reported to be observed within the first 6 days of symptoms.[28] In a retrospective study that analyzed SARS-CoV-2 transmission in household contacts, the Ct value of the index cases was independently associated with the risk of secondary attacks. However, viral transmission was detectable among at least 20% of all and 40% of tested household contacts when index cases had Ct values more than 31,[29] highlighting significant limitations of using a cutoff of 30 cycles for infection control decisions and using cell culture to estimate infectiousness. The same group demonstrated, in a follow-up study, that the initial inoculum and the index case Ct value do not associate with the disease outcome of the secondary cases.[30] Separate research that used undergraduate students' surveillance data showed that the Ct values could not predict the transmissibility and an overlap was seen in the Ct value ranges observed in those who were identified as spreaders and non-spreaders.[31] Of note, the study cohort spanned the time frame between September 2020 and October 2020, which was before the rollout of vaccination. The data indicate that Ct values might predict a higher likelihood of recovering infectious virus but cannot reliably predict transmissibility.

What Is the Impact of Viral Evolution?

SARS-CoV-2 has continued to evolve since its first emergence in 2019, and novel variants have raised continuous concerns about potential increased infectiousness and transmissibility. With every wave of new variants, the mean Ct values of new positive samples drop, correlating with an increased transmission of the novel variant,[32,33] which might imply a direct relation between viral loads and variants spread. The Delta variant showed a reduced average Ct value when compared with Alpha and demonstrated an increased recovery of infectious virus in cell culture.[19] That being said, the correlation between Ct values and the recovery of infectious virus differed among various SARS-CoV-2 variants.[34] Specifically, the Omicron variant, which led to an unprecedented increase in transmissibility and disease prevalence, exhibited a less successful recovery in cell culture compared with Delta, despite having similar average Ct values in newly infected patients.[18,35] In contrast to Delta, the recovery of Omicron in cell culture was not influenced by prior vaccinations,[18,36] suggesting that the overall rise in Omicron transmissibility was more likely associated with immune evasion. This suggests that Ct values and the infectious virus load, as determined by cell culture, are insufficient to explain the heightened transmissibility of Omicron and raises doubts about the usefulness of Ct values as a predictive factor for infectiousness when novel variants emerge. Preexisting immune responses resulting from prior infections or vaccination likely played a substantial role in the kinetics of viral shedding and transmissibility during each wave of variants.

Can Rapid Antigen Detection Be Used as a Proxy for Infectiousness?

Lateral flow assays, used for rapid SARS-CoV-2 antigen detection, were evaluated as a proxy for infectiousness, and a relationship was observed between antigen positivity, Ct values, and the recovery of infectious virus.[37–39] The lower sensitivity of antigen tests, particularly when Ct values exceed 25, accounts for the agreement with cell culture isolations. Antigen tests yield the highest positive results within the initial 7 days of symptom onset,[40] and the first positive result might be delayed compared with the first molecular result. Importantly, negative antigen results have been reported in samples containing infectious virus or with low Ct values,[41] and viral mutations that impacted their sensitivity were identified.[42,43] In a human challenge study, the detection of infectious virus occurred one or more days before the initial positive antigen detection.[44] This finding aligns with another retrospective study, which indicated that the sensitivity of antigen testing was only 50% during the presumed infectious period.[45] Taken together, antigen testing shares the same limitations as using Ct values as a measure of infectiousness and encounters additional challenges due to its low sensitivity (**Boxes 1** and **2**).

Severe Acute Respiratory Syndrome Coronavirus 2 (SARS-CoV-2) Subgenomic RNAs

SARS-CoV-2 possesses a positive-sense RNA genome that undergoes replication by transcribing its genome into negative-sense RNA intermediate strands. These negative-sense strands then serve as templates for the production of positive-sense genomic RNA. Discontinuous transcription leads to the generation of sgRNAs that contain transcription-regulating sequences situated at the end of the leader sequence within the 5′ untranslated region,[55] and their detection would likely indicate active viral replication and, consequently, infectiousness. However, it was found that the Ct values of genomic RNA and sgRNA exhibited a strong correlation, and the effectiveness of sgRNA in predicting replicating virus was limited.[56] In a study on prolonged SARS-CoV-2 shedding, sgRNA was detected in 20% of patients between 28 and 79 days after symptom onset.[57] Another research group demonstrated that sgRNAs were shielded by cellular membranes, raising doubts about their effectiveness as an active replication

Box 1
Limitations of viral load estimation using cycle threshold values

- Ct values are generated by qualitatively developed assays and cannot be relied on as a surrogate measure of viral load.
- Several variables can influence Ct values and, more significantly, pose challenges to their comparability across various assays and laboratories.
- These variables include specimen type, sample collection, collection media, sample transport and storage conditions, sample volume, selected gene targets, primers and probes, and any mutations that may affect their binding sites, as well as extraction methods, among others.[9]
- Achieving comparability between assays is only feasible when calibration and standardization of genomic quantification are based on universal standards.
- That said, published studies showed some value for using Ct values in disease prognosis, predicting disease trends and surveillance, patients' management, and infection control.[11,46–50]

Box 2
Limitations of cell culture for recovering infectious virus

- Virus isolation using specific cell lines has been widely regarded as the most accepted method for determining the presence of infectious virus particles, considered the gold standard.
- Various cell lines, including Vero E6 and those expressing angiotensin-converting enzyme 2 (ACE-2) and/or transmembrane protease 2, have been used for isolating SARS-CoV-2.[1,18,19,51]
- Different studies have used distinct cell lines and incubation times, potentially contributing to discrepancies in the sensitivity of viral isolation.
- Variables beyond Ct values can influence the isolation of infectious virus in cell culture, such as sample integrity, storage conditions,[52] and the presence of neutralizing antibodies.[53]
- It is important to note that SARS-CoV-2 cell culture experiments can currently only be conducted under strict biosafety level 3 (BSL-3) conditions, significantly limiting its applicability.
- Generally, cell culture for viral isolation is insensitive and the time to results is extended, challenging its clinical utility.[54]

marker.[58] When compared with antigen testing, the overall agreement was 92%, and 84.8% of samples positive for negative-sense RNA tested negative for the isolation of infectious virus in cell culture.[59] In an effort to aid clinical decision-making and infection control for chronically infected patients, a strand-specific reverse transcriptase quantitative polymerase chain reaction (PCR) assay was developed as an alternative to sgRNA detection.[60] This assay was capable of detecting the negative-sense RNA intermediate for up to 30 days after symptom onset. Collectively, these findings suggest that the utility of sgRNA and negative-strand RNA detection is limited in predicting infectiousness.

Future Directions

Even though the COVID-19 pandemic was associated with an unprecedented evolution of viral diagnostics using various technologies that offered a wide range of sensitivities, no assays were developed to specifically identify infectious individuals. Various approaches were taken to estimate infectiousness, including primarily Ct values, however, proper clinical validations that support clinical cutoffs are lacking, imposing significant diagnostic stewardship issues. Evidence and published data, even though, can support epidemiologic utility, they can't endorse individual level clinical decisions. Identifying the minimum infective dose might facilitate the validation of cutoff viral loads below which patients would be less likely to be infectious. However, standardizing methods for viral quantification and specifying the minimum infective dose is needed to facilitate clinical interpretations. A human challenge study showed that infecting volunteer individuals, who were not previously vaccinated and without evidence of prior infection, with 10 TCID50 of a SARS-CoV-2 original viral strain resulted in a confirmed infection in 18 out of a total of 34.[44] Observational studies suggested that the minimum infective dose of SARS-CoV-2 is low and varies by age.[61] These observations highlight the significant contribution of host factors to susceptibility to infection and the complexity of identifying a viral minimum infective dose. Approaches that can directly detect infectious virus particles in patients' samples with high sensitivity and a quick turnaround are urgently needed. SARS-CoV-2 Spike-ACE-2 binding assays were developed for evaluating and quantifying neutralizing antibodies and for screening for SARS-CoV-2 inhibitors.[62] These assays are based on the interaction between the SARS-CoV-2 spike protein and ACE-2 and have used recombinant proteins and ELISA-based approaches. Such an interaction was also successfully detected in living cells using time-resolved fluorescence resonance energy transfer.[63] Leveraging such a concept for detecting infectious virus in patients' samples can be a promising direct approach for testing for infectiousness.

DISCLOSURES

The author declares no relevant competing interests. H.H. Mostafa received honoraria from BD Diagnostics and Bio-Rad, has research collaborations with Qiagen, Bio-Rad, and Hologic, and serves on the advisory committee of Seegene.

REFERENCES

1. Gniazdowski V, Paul Morris C, Wohl S, et al. Repeated Coronavirus Disease 2019 Molecular Testing: Correlation of Severe Acute Respiratory Syndrome Coronavirus 2 Culture With Molecular Assays and Cycle Thresholds. Clin Infect Dis 2021;73(4):e860–9.
2. He X, Lau EHY, Wu P, et al. Temporal dynamics in viral shedding and transmissibility of COVID-19. Nat Med 2020;26(5):672–5.
3. Wolfel R, Corman VM, Guggemos W, et al. Virological assessment of hospitalized patients with COVID-2019. Nature 2020;581(7809):465–9.
4. Gombar S, Chang M, Hogan CA, et al. Persistent detection of SARS-CoV-2 RNA in patients and healthcare workers with COVID-19. J Clin Virol 2020;129:104477.
5. Fleury H, Burrel S, Balick Weber C, et al. Prolonged shedding of influenza A(H1N1)v virus: two case reports from France 2009. Euro Surveill 2009;14(49):19434.
6. Wang Y, Guo Q, Yan Z, et al. Factors associated with prolonged viral shedding in patients with avian influenza A(H7N9) virus infection. J Infect Dis 2018;217(11):1708–17.
7. Zlateva KT, de Vries JJ, Coenjaerts FE, et al. Prolonged shedding of rhinovirus and re-infection in adults with respiratory tract illness. Eur Respir J 2014;44(1):169–77.
8. Leung NHL. Transmissibility and transmission of respiratory viruses. Nat Rev Microbiol 2021;19(8):528–45.
9. Rhoads D, Peaper DR, She RC, et al. College of American pathologists (CAP) microbiology committee perspective: caution must Be used in interpreting the cycle threshold (Ct) value. Clin Infect Dis 2021;72(10):e685–6.
10. Goyal P, Choi JJ, Pinheiro LC, et al. Clinical characteristics of covid-19 in New York city. N Engl J Med 2020;382(24):2372–4.
11. Dioverti MV, Gaston DC, Morris CP, et al. Combination Therapy With Casirivimab/Imdevimab and Remdesivir for Protracted SARS-CoV-2 Infection in B-cell-Depleted Patients. Open Forum Infect Dis 2022;9(6):ofac064.
12. Mowrer CT, Creager H, Cawcutt K, et al. Evaluation of cycle threshold values at deisolation. Infect Control Hosp Epidemiol 2022;43(6):794–6.
13. Tu Y-P, Iqbal J, O'Leary T. Sensitivity of ID NOW and RT–PCR for detection of SARS-CoV-2 in an ambulatory population. Elife 2021;10:e65726.
14. Platten M, Hoffmann D, Grosser R, et al. SARS-CoV-2, CT-Values, and Infectivity-Conclusions to Be Drawn from Side Observations. Viruses 2021;13(8):1459.
15. Brandolini M, Taddei F, Marino MM, et al. Correlating qRT-PCR, dPCR and Viral Titration for the Identification and Quantification of SARS-CoV-2: A New Approach for Infection Management. Viruses 2021;13(6):1022.

16. Gniazdowski V, Paul Morris C, Wohl S, et al. Repeated coronavirus disease 2019 molecular testing: correlation of severe acute respiratory syndrome coronavirus 2 culture with molecular assays and cycle thresholds. Clin Infect Dis 2021;73(4): e860–9.
17. Singanayagam A, Patel M, Charlett A, et al. Duration of infectiousness and correlation with RT-PCR cycle threshold values in cases of COVID-19, England, January to May 2020. Euro Surveill 2020;25(32):2001483.
18. Fall A, Eldesouki RE, Sachithanandham J, et al. The displacement of the SARS-CoV-2 variant Delta with Omicron: an investigation of hospital admissions and upper respiratory viral loads. EBioMedicine 2022;79:104008.
19. Huai Luo C, Paul Morris C, Sachithanandham J, et al. Infection with the severe acute respiratory syndrome coronavirus 2 (SARS-CoV-2) Delta variant is associated with higher recovery of infectious virus compared to the Alpha variant in both unvaccinated and vaccinated individuals. Clin Infect Dis 2022;75(1):e715–25.
20. Mostafa HH, Luo CH, Morris CP, et al. SARS-CoV-2 infections in mRNA vaccinated individuals are biased for viruses encoding spike E484K and associated with reduced infectious virus loads that correlate with respiratory antiviral IgG levels. J Clin Virol 2022;150-151:105151.
21. Yang Y, Guo L, Yuan J, et al. Viral and antibody dynamics of acute infection with SARS-CoV-2 omicron variant (B.1.1.529): a prospective cohort study from Shenzhen, China. Lancet Microbe 2023;4(8):e632–41.
22. Frediani JK, Parsons R, McLendon KB, et al. The New Normal: Delayed Peak SARS-CoV-2 Viral Loads Relative to Symptom Onset and Implications for COVID-19 Testing Programs. Clin Infect Dis 2023;ciad582.
23. Morris CP, Luo CH, Sachithanandham J, et al. Large Scale SARS-CoV-2 Molecular Testing and Genomic Surveillance Reveal Prolonged Infections, Protracted RNA shedding, and Viral Reinfections. Front Cell Infect Microbiol 2022;12: 809407.
24. van der Vries E, Stittelaar KJ, van Amerongen G, et al. Prolonged influenza virus shedding and emergence of antiviral resistance in immunocompromised patients and ferrets. PLoS Pathog 2013;9(5):e1003343.
25. de Lima CR, Mirandolli TB, Carneiro LC, et al. Prolonged respiratory viral shedding in transplant patients. Transpl Infect Dis 2014;16(1):165–9.
26. Lehners N, Tabatabai J, Prifert C, et al. Long-term shedding of influenza virus, parainfluenza virus, respiratory syncytial virus and nosocomial epidemiology in patients with hematological disorders. PLoS One 2016;11(2):e0148258.
27. Marks M, Millat-Martinez P, Ouchi D, et al. Transmission of COVID-19 in 282 clusters in Catalonia, Spain: a cohort study. Lancet Infect Dis 2021;21(5):629–36.
28. Cheng HY, Jian SW, Liu DP, et al. Contact tracing assessment of COVID-19 transmission dynamics in Taiwan and risk at different exposure periods before and after symptom onset. JAMA Intern Med 2020;180(9):1156–63.
29. Trunfio M, Richiardi L, Alladio F, et al. Determinants of SARS-CoV-2 Contagiousness in Household Contacts of Symptomatic Adult Index Cases. Front Microbiol 2022;13:829393.
30. Trunfio M, Longo BM, Alladio F, et al. On the SARS-CoV-2 "variolation hypothesis": No association between viral load of index cases and COVID-19 severity of secondary cases. Front Microbiol 2021;12:646679.
31. Tian D, Lin Z, Kriner EM, et al. Ct values do not predict severe acute respiratory syndrome coronavirus 2 (SARS-CoV-2) transmissibility in college students. J Mol Diagn 2021;23(9):1078–84.

32. Sala E, Shah IS, Manissero D, et al. Systematic review on the correlation between SARS-CoV-2 real-time PCR cycle threshold values and epidemiological trends. Infect Dis Ther 2023;12(3):749–75.
33. Walker AS, Pritchard E, House T, et al. Ct threshold values, a proxy for viral load in community SARS-CoV-2 cases, demonstrate wide variation across populations and over time. Elife 2021;10:e64683.
34. Tassetto M, Garcia-Knight M, Anglin K, et al. Detection of higher cycle threshold values in culturable SARS-CoV-2 omicron BA.1 sublineage compared with pre-omicron variant specimens - San Francisco bay area, California July 2021-march 2022. MMWR Morb Mortal Wkly Rep 2022;71(36):1151–4.
35. Bordoy AE, Saludes V, Panisello Yagüe D, et al. Monitoring SARS-CoV-2 variant transitions using differences in diagnostic cycle threshold values of target genes. Sci Rep 2022;12(1):21818.
36. Puhach O, Adea K, Hulo N, et al. Infectious viral load in unvaccinated and vaccinated individuals infected with ancestral, Delta or Omicron SARS-CoV-2. Nat Med 2022;28(7):1491–500.
37. Kirby JE, Riedel S, Dutta S, et al. Sars-Cov-2 antigen tests predict infectivity based on viral culture: comparison of antigen, PCR viral load, and viral culture testing on a large sample cohort. Clin Microbiol Infection 2023;29(1):94–100.
38. Pickering S, Batra R, Merrick B, et al. Comparative performance of SARS-CoV-2 lateral flow antigen tests and association with detection of infectious virus in clinical specimens: a single-centre laboratory evaluation study. Lancet Microbe 2021;2(9):e461–71.
39. Korenkov M, Poopalasingam N, Madler M, et al. Evaluation of a rapid antigen test to detect SARS-CoV-2 infection and identify potentially infectious individuals. J Clin Microbiol 2021;59(9):e0089621.
40. Dinnes J, Sharma P, Berhane S, et al. Rapid, point-of-care antigen tests for diagnosis of SARS-CoV-2 infection. Cochrane Database Syst Rev 2022;7(7): Cd013705.
41. Currie DW, Shah MM, Salvatore PP, et al. Relationship of SARS-CoV-2 antigen and reverse transcription PCR positivity for viral cultures. Emerg Infect Dis 2022;28(3):717–20.
42. Frank F, Keen MM, Rao A, et al. Deep mutational scanning identifies SARS-CoV-2 Nucleocapsid escape mutations of currently available rapid antigen tests. Cell 2022;185(19):3603–16.e3613.
43. Del Vecchio C, Cracknell Daniels B, Brancaccio G, et al. Impact of antigen test target failure and testing strategies on the transmission of SARS-CoV-2 variants. Nat Commun 2022;13(1):5870.
44. Killingley B, Mann AJ, Kalinova M, et al. Safety, tolerability and viral kinetics during SARS-CoV-2 human challenge in young adults. Nat Med 2022;28(5):1031–41.
45. Chu VT, Schwartz NG, Donnelly MAP, et al. Comparison of home antigen testing with RT-PCR and viral culture during the course of SARS-CoV-2 infection. JAMA Intern Med 2022;182(7):701–9.
46. Westblade LF, Brar G, Pinheiro LC, et al. SARS-CoV-2 viral load predicts mortality in patients with and without cancer who are hospitalized with COVID-19. Cancer Cell 2020;38(5):661–71.e662.
47. Magleby R, Westblade LF, Trzebucki A, et al. Impact of severe acute respiratory syndrome coronavirus 2 viral load on risk of intubation and mortality among hospitalized patients with coronavirus disease 2019. Clin Infect Dis 2021;73(11): e4197–205.

48. Shah VP, Farah WH, Hill JC, et al. Association between SARS-CoV-2 cycle threshold values and clinical outcomes in patients with COVID-19: a systematic review and meta-analysis. Open Forum Infect Dis 2021;8(9):ofab453.
49. Satlin MJ, Zucker J, Baer BR, et al. Changes in SARS-CoV-2 viral load and mortality during the initial wave of the pandemic in New York City. PLoS One 2021; 16(11):e0257979.
50. Rodino KG, Peaper DR, Kelly BJ, et al. Partial ORF1ab gene target failure with omicron BA.2.12.1. J Clin Microbiol 2022;60(6):e00600–22.
51. Morris CP, Eldesouki RE, Sachithanandham J, et al. Omicron subvariants: clinical, laboratory, and cell culture characterization. Clin Infect Dis 2023;76(7):1276–84.
52. Huang C-G, Lee K-M, Hsiao M-J, et al. Culture-based virus isolation to evaluate potential infectivity of clinical specimens tested for COVID-19. J Clin Microbiol 2020;58(8). https://doi.org/10.1128/jcm.01068-01020.
53. Atkinson B, Petersen E. SARS-CoV-2 shedding and infectivity. Lancet 2020; 395(10233):1339–40.
54. Hodinka RL. Point: is the era of viral culture over in the clinical microbiology laboratory? J Clin Microbiol 2013;51(1):2–4.
55. Long S. SARS-CoV-2 Subgenomic RNAs: Characterization, Utility, and Perspectives. Viruses 2021;13(10):1923.
56. Roesmann F, Jakobsche I, Pallas C, et al. Comparison of the Ct-values for genomic and subgenomic SARS-CoV-2 RNA reveals limited predictive value for the presence of replication competent virus. J Clin Virol 2023;165:105499.
57. Rodríguez-Grande C, Adán-Jiménez J, Catalán P, et al. Inference of Active Viral Replication in Cases with Sustained Positive Reverse Transcription-PCR Results for SARS-CoV-2. J Clin Microbiol 2021;59(2):e02277–20.
58. Alexandersen S, Chamings A, Bhatta TR. SARS-CoV-2 genomic and subgenomic RNAs in diagnostic samples are not an indicator of active replication. Nat Commun 2020;11(1):6059.
59. Chang-Graham AL, Sahoo MK, Huang C, et al. Comparison of nucleocapsid antigen with strand-specific reverse-transcription PCR for monitoring SARS-CoV-2 infection. J Clin Virol 2023;164:105468.
60. Hogan CA, Huang C, Sahoo MK, et al. Strand-specific reverse transcription PCR for detection of replicating SARS-CoV-2. Emerg Infect Dis 2021;27(2):632–5.
61. SeyedAlinaghi S, Karimi A, Mojdeganlou H, et al. Minimum infective dose of severe acute respiratory syndrome coronavirus 2 based on the current evidence: a systematic review. SAGE Open Med 2022;10:20503121221115053.
62. Zhang S, Gao C, Das T, et al. The spike-ACE2 binding assay: an in vitro platform for evaluating vaccination efficacy and for screening SARS-CoV-2 inhibitors and neutralizing antibodies. J Immunol Methods 2022;503:113244.
63. Cecon E, Dam J, Jockers R. Detection of SARS-CoV-2 spike protein binding to ACE2 in living cells by TR-FRET. STAR Protoc 2022;3(1):101024.

Working with the Electronic Health Record and Laboratory Information System to Maximize Ordering and Reporting of Molecular Microbiology Results

Meghan W. Starolis, PhD[a,*], Mark A. Zaydman, MD, PhD[b], Rachael M. Liesman, PhD[c]

KEYWORDS

- Laboratory information systems • Electronic health records
- Laboratory stewardship • Molecular microbiology • Infectious disease

KEY POINTS

- Preanalytical tools, such as best practice alerts or evidence-based order guidelines, can be deployed for improved laboratory stewardship of high-cost molecular microbiology testing.
- Postanalytical tools can be utilized for proper result interpretation and appropriate follow-up.
- Emerging technologies such as artificial intelligence and machine learning have the potential to be used in clinical practice for both stewardship and clinical decision support.

INTRODUCTION

The evolution and availability of nucleic acid amplification techniques (NAATs) such as polymerase chain reaction (PCR) have significantly changed infectious disease testing beyond the traditional microbiology paradigm.[1] Today, molecular assays can be found routinely in laboratories of varying Clinical Laboratory Improvement Amendments (CLIA) complexity, with many that are Food and Drug Administration (FDA)–approved or CLIA-waived. Additionally, emerging technologies are aiming to change

[a] Molecular Infectious Disease, Quest Diagnostics, 14225 Newbrook Drive, Chantilly, VA 20151, USA; [b] Department of Pathology & Immunology, Washington University School of Medicine, Campus Box 8118, 660 South Euclid Avenue, St Louis, MO 63110, USA; [c] Clinical Microbiology and Molecular Diagnostics Pathology, Department of Pathology, Medical College of Wisconsin, 9200 West Wisconsin, Milwaukee, WI 53226, USA
* Corresponding author.
E-mail address: meghan.w.starolis@questdiagnostics.com

Clin Lab Med 44 (2024) 95–107
https://doi.org/10.1016/j.cll.2023.10.009

the "one assay, one organism" testing approach. For example, the ability to multiplex (ie, multiple targets detected in a single reaction) has led to the development of syndromic panels for conditions such as gastroenteritis, respiratory illness, sepsis, and joint infections.[2] Advanced amplification techniques such as targeted and metagenomic next-generation sequencing are capable of detecting hundreds of organisms.[3] With these advances has come a substantial increase in the cost of testing compared to traditional methods owing to the high cost of reagents (primers, probes, enzymes, master mix) and instrumentation such as thermocyclers and sequencers. The cost and unclear clinical utility of some tests warrant laboratory stewardship, and there is often a disconnect between the ordering physician and laboratorians.[4]

In addition to managing costs, a successful laboratory stewardship program must endeavor to reduce medical errors, improve test utilization, improve diagnostic accuracy, and support antibiotic stewardship. There are often clinical practice guidelines for infectious conditions and nuances associated with laboratory testing and interpretation of specific pathogens. It is unreasonable to expect physicians of varying specialties to be familiar with the myriad of best practices for infectious disease diagnosis, and while clinicians should utilize the expertise of their laboratory director, the capabilities of electronic tools to influence ordering practices must also be leveraged. We will discuss ways that tools in the electronic health record (EHR), and laboratory information system (LIS) and future tools such as artificial intelligence (AI) and machine learning (ML) can be used for laboratory stewardship of these methods.

THE 'DIGITAL LIFE CYCLE' OF A LABORATORY TEST

The process of ordering laboratory tests and receiving results has changed radically as paper-based and fax-based ordering processes have given way to electronic user interfaces connected to computerized systems. As a result, new opportunities are available to integrate electronic utilization management tools and clinical decision support (CDS) as information flows digitally through preanalytical, analytical, and postanalytical phases of the testing process. As summarized in **Fig. 1**, information is passed between several electronic systems, including the computerized physician order entry (CPOE), EHR, LIS, middleware, and the laboratory analyzer throughout the testing process. Each system serves a specific purpose, contains distinct sets of information, and presents unique opportunities for utilization management and CDS.

Computerized Physician Order Entry

CPOE is a software application enabling qualified individuals to enter orders that trigger downstream actions in the testing process. The CPOE is often an integrated EHR module and is the main interface for the ordering provider. This integration provides real-time access to clinical information including diagnoses, imaging studies, provider notes, prescriptions, and medication administrations. These attributes make the CPOE a particularly useful environment for utilization management interventions.

An attractive feature of CPOE-based interventions is that they are timely and occur while the user is actively engaged in resolving test utilization decisions for the patient.

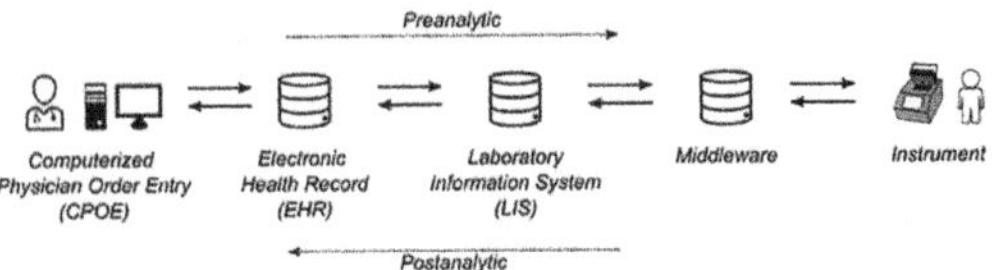

Fig. 1. Information systems involved in the generation of a laboratory result.

Later interventions may be less likely to succeed due to anchoring biases and limited time for revisiting prior decisions. In addition, intervention at the point of order precedes specimen collection, thus minimizing patient discomfort. Additionally, CDS at the point of order entry may guide the selection and timely performance of an appropriate alternative test that might have been otherwise missed. A major drawback of EHR/CPOE-based interventions is that they can add to the work of the order entry user, potentially contributing to fatigue and burnout among health care professionals.[5] For this reason, EHR/CPOE-based interventions should be carefully designed to minimize disruption and reevaluated after deployment to identify and eliminate low-value interventions. For example, review of CPOE pop-up alert data, formalized alert governance, stakeholder engagement, and alert optimization through the '5 rights of CDS' (right information, right person, right time, right channel, and right format)[6] led to a ~60% decrease in the total alert volume and a significant increase in the acceptance rates from 8% to 54.7%.[7]

A limitation of CPOE-based interventions is that the individual entering the order may not be the individual to whom the CDS intervention is targeted. In a study of the effectiveness of a pop-up alert designed to reduce unnecessary repetitive testing within a single patient encounter, compliance rates were significantly higher for attending physicians (62.8%) versus nurses (22.9%).[8] These results suggest that the effectiveness of the CPOE-based interventions may be limited by the degree to which the CPOE user feels empowered to make care decisions. Another limitation is that some testing workflows such as point-of-care molecular testing engage the CPOE only after testing for result entry into the EHR.

Laboratory Information System

The LIS is a software application that helps to manage laboratory workflows and operations. The scope of the data within the LIS partially overlaps with that in the EHR. Specifically, the LIS captures basic patient demographics, billing data, laboratory orders, and specimen collection information. However, much of the clinical data related to diagnoses, histories, clinical observations, and medications does not flow across the EHR to the LIS interface. Additionally, because the ordering provider does not typically interact with the LIS, there are fewer opportunities to provide patient-specific interventions. The LIS does have unique data elements, such as preliminary laboratory results, reagent availability, specimen inventories, and quality control data, which can be leveraged to steer utilization. An attractive attribute of LIS-based strategies is that they occur in the background from the perspective of the ordering provider and do not impact their workflows. An example of a LIS-based utilization management intervention is reflexive testing algorithms, for example, automated ordering of a human immunodeficiency virus (HIV)–genotyping assay based on positive HIV NAAT results with sufficient viral load. The major drawback is limited intervention personalization due to lack of access to the clinical data within the EHR. This limitation may be addressed as institutions adopt data warehousing strategies (data repositories that centralize data from different sources).[9]

Middleware

Middleware is a software application that sits between the LIS and the laboratory analyzer (when applicable). Middleware can be used to extend the functionality of the LIS and can serve as a common adapter to multiple instruments and automation lines. Middleware provides opportunities to integrate testing and verification logic that might trigger additional or repeat testing (eg, repeat on 10x dilution if the result is greater than linearity). While these middleware processes may seem far removed from the clinician, they are a form of utilization management as the ordering provider does not have to order repeat testing. Ideally, these process control points would occur proximal to the point and time of testing while the specimen is still on or near the analyzer. Additionally, verification logic can trigger result comments or flags for abnormality or critical results. These middleware actions guide the clinician's interpretation in the postanalytical phase of the test cycle.

Instrument (Laboratory Analyzer)

The laboratory analyzer is controlled by a dedicated set of computer hardware and software that are typically vendor supported. A unique opportunity at the laboratory analyzer level is access to the raw data and reaction monitoring. These granular data exist only on the analyzer, as transmitting and storing it in the LIS would be expensive. Therefore, if the assay characteristics (eg, cycle threshold [Ct] values, relative light units) are relevant to utilization management or interpretation, the instrument may be a logical intervention point.

DISCUSSION

Preanaltyical Tools

CDS is most often implemented at the point of ordering in the preanalytic testing phase. Preanalytical CDS can take many forms, including best practice alerts (BPAs), test restrictions, automated reflex testing, and establishing testing algorithms, order sets, or panels. Effective test utilization initiatives often require the implementation of multiple strategies.

Best practice alerts

BPAs are automated interruptive alerts that appear, or "fire," within the EHR at a defined point, such as on test order placement. BPAs are a common approach to CPOE-based CDS and often prompt a specific action (eg, ordering a test, acknowledging the alert). Alerts can be grouped into 3 categories: hard stop, soft stop, and passive. Soft-stop BPAs are considered nudges, a term that describes providing choices that encourage a specific outcome while preserving the freedom of choice.[10] The user is allowed to proceed with the initial choice by acknowledging and overriding the alert. Hard-stop BPAs force a specific action by preventing the override process. Passive alerts provide information but do not require user interaction or interrupt the clinical workflow. Within the scope of molecular diagnostic stewardship, alerts may be used to increase ordering of screening tests, prevent duplicative ordering, and reduce utilization of expensive or inappropriate tests.[8,11–13]

To prevent or reduce repeat ordering for costly or frequently overutilized molecular tests, laboratories may establish test-specific minimum retesting intervals (MRI), defined as "the minimum time before a test should be repeated based on the properties of the test and the clinical situation in which it is used," and implement BPAs on tests ordered within the MRI.[14] For example, hard-stop BPAs have been used to restrict repeat orders of multiplex NAATs for respiratory pathogens within a specified time frame due to minimal clinical utility within 20 days of previous testing.[15] Another study showed that use of a multiplex gastrointestinal (GI) panel in patients hospitalized greater than 3 days yielded clinically actionable data in only 3% (12/406) of cases.[16] Repeat GI panel testing within 4 weeks of an initial negative test yielded a positive result in 7.6% (11/145) of cases, suggesting limited clinical utility of repeat testing within this interval.[17] Similarly, within 7 days of an initial negative *Clostridium difficile* NAAT, 1% to 3.3% of tests yielded a positive result upon repeat testing and implementation of a CPOE-based alert within this timeframe reduced inappropriate repeat testing by 91% in 1 institution.[12,18]

Physicians may be unaware of the cost of certain diagnostic tests and disclosing those costs at the time of ordering may facilitate sensible use of expensive or poorly reimbursed tests. A study of fee data displayed within the CPOE system demonstrated a modest reduction in tests ordered.[19] Such an intervention may be implemented for expensive molecular tests, such as multiplex panels or sequencing-based tests, although the efficacy of these interventions may be enhanced by pairing with other utilization strategies. For example, one intervention aimed to reduce use of a multiplex molecular respiratory viral panel (RVP) by implementing 2 noninterruptive CDS strategies.[20] First, the test cost and indication for appropriate use were disclosed by adding a message to the test display name. Second, EHR order search synonyms such as "virus," "flu," and "RSV" were removed from the RVP order so that when providers searched using these terms, only the influenza/respiratory syncytial virus (RSV) order would display. Postimplementation, RVP orders were 71% lower than in the preimplementation period, demonstrating that noninterruptive CDS strategies can successfully modify ordering behavior.

BPAs can incorporate other laboratory or clinical data to recommend ordering changes in specific clinical scenarios. Soft-stop BPAs are increasingly used to optimize *C difficile* testing to reduce the overtreatment of patients who are colonized but do not have disease. In 1 study, implementation of a BPA to alert the ordering provider that a patient had recent use of a laxative or stool softeners led to a 21% reduction in inappropriate *C difficile* orders.[21] Hamilton and colleagues developed a decision tree algorithm using basic laboratory data (white blood cell and liver function tests) to support appropriate use of *Anaplasma* molecular testing, demonstrating that the proposed criteria would reduce unnecessary testing by 21%.[22] Finally, order-associated questions, sometimes called "ask at order entry questions," can capture data elements not easily extractable from the EHR to support more complex interventions. A tertiary care hospital developed CPOE-based decision support for *C difficile* testing via a 2-step tool incorporating order-associated questions.[23] The first alert detected duplicate testing within a 28-day timeframe. The second tool included a series of yes/no questions designed to identify tests ordered outside of evidence-based practice guidelines. If testing was deemed inappropriate based on answers to the prompts, the provider received an alert recommending test cancellation with the option to either cancel the order or override the alert. Postimplementation analysis demonstrated a 41% reduction in test volume with no change in overall test positivity.

Despite some evidence of success, the efficacy of BPAs varies significantly by study, with many suggesting BPAs are often overridden and ineffective. Providers report feeling "alert fatigue" when inundated with alerts and clicks within the EHR which can ultimately lead to ignoring the information provided in the alert.[24] Additionally, the information in the BPA may be insufficient to overcome protocolized behavior or clinical inertia. Ultimately, BPAs may be more effective at eliciting an action rather than preventing one, and those aimed at reducing inappropriate testing may be most effective when paired with additional interventions. To support this, an analysis of 51 studies in health care settings demonstrated that use of multiple nudges concurrently increased the likelihood of effective behavior modification.[10] Hard-stop BPAs are more effective than those that allow an override option but are often viewed unfavorable by physicians. A direct comparison of a hard-stopto soft-stop BPA for the reduction of duplicate testing demonstrated a 92.3% reduction in duplicate orders when implementing a hard-stop, while a soft-stop reduced duplicate orders by 42.6%.[25] Because a hard-stop BPA does not allow for dismissal, these should be used judiciously, and physicians should be informed of the process for overriding the BPA, when appropriate, to avoid delays to patient care.[26]

Gatekeeping

Gatekeeping, or test restriction, is a strategy generally aimed at preventing test overutilization. For example, implementation of age-based white blood cell count restriction criteria in cerebrospinal fluid (CSF) samples with an order for a meningitis/encephalitis (M/E) NAAT panel reduced panel utilization by 42.7%.[27] However, most gatekeeping strategies require a manual chart review by a pathology resident or a medical director which can limit the scalability and sustainability of this strategy. Gatekeeping may be electronically deployed by restricting tests to specific provider subspecialties or locations (eg, inpatient vs ambulatory) or implementing a reflex algorithm strategy to restrict test ordering unless other criteria are met. Laboratory tests that are rarely appropriate based on evidence-based guidelines should be removed from the laboratory test formulary.

Order sets

An order set is a group of pretemplated orders used to standardize and expedite the ordering process. Standardized order sets are an important CPOE-based CDS tool and may be developed based on clinical indication (eg, acute diarrhea) or patient encounter type (eg, an admission order set). Order sets may be designed as an opt-in (no tests are preselected), opt-out (all tests are preselected), or a combination of the two where only recommended tests are preselected. Because incorporation of tests into order sets may increase inappropriate use due to nonspecific ordering practices, utilization monitoring following order set updates is recommended.[28] In 1 such example, NAATs for the detection of viral pathogens in the central nervous system (CNS) (herpes simplex virus [HSV], varicella zoster virus, cytomegalovirus, and enterovirus [EV]) were incorporated into an inpatient order set, leading to a 54% to 62% increase in test ordering.[13] However, increased ordering was associated with an 11% relative decrease in NAAT positivity, suggesting that implementation of the order set did not improve detection of viral CNS infections. When testing was restricted to patients meeting acceptance criteria (all immunosuppressed patients and immunocompetent patients with CSF white blood count>10 cells/μl) in addition to seasonal restriction of EV testing (April to October), a 46% reduction in orders was observed.

Reflex testing and order panels

Laboratories often develop algorithms to align with guideline-based ordering recommendations. Some algorithms may include reflex testing, where a test is automatically performed after an initial test based on predetermined criteria such as hepatitis C virus (HCV) NAAT for confirmation of HCV antibody testing.[29] Reflex testing algorithms do not require additional physician orders or specimen collection, supporting a shorter turnaround time and preventing misutilization of downstream confirmatory tests. Reflex testing that is not required by regulatory standards must be approved by a medical executive committee to ensure alignment with best available practices and should be disclosed to the ordering physician.[30]

Algorithm-based testing strategies that do not include reflex testing may include order panels, also known as order profiles. Order panels are a battery of individual tests that are grouped under a unique name. Order panels may require all tests within the panel to be run or a subset chosen by the ordering provider. For example, a seasonal virus panel may offer the option of various combinations of influenza virus, severe acute respiratory syndrome coronavirus 2, and RSV testing within the order panel. Regulatory compliance requires that most tests offered within panels also be offered individually.

Postanalytical Tools

While the best opportunity for electronic tools to contribute to diagnostic stewardship is before the order has been placed, there are significant opportunities postanalytically to encourage health care stewardship. Several postanalytical tools including flagging of abnormal results, canned comments, and nudges can optimize physician time, expedite result review and interpretation, and encourage appropriate follow-up.

Flagging abnormal results

Flagging of abnormal results is programmed into the reporting system based on predefined rules and helps the physician to identify clinically actionable results faster. It is advisable to use more than 1 flagging strategy to accommodate different functionality in EHRs. Examples include the use of color coding (eg, green for normal results, red for abnormal results), moving abnormal results to an 'out of range' column, and use of an asterisk or letter beside the abnormal result ("L" or "H" flags [low/high], "C" [critical], "A" [abnormal]). Any abnormal result should be flagged but careful attention should be paid to the detection of microorganisms in sterile body sites (eg, CSF) and those that cause life-threatening diseases.[31] Examples would be detection of any microorganism using a molecular syndromic M/E panel or blood culture identification (BCID) panel as these results are time-critical for patient management. Unfortunately, no standard flagging convention exists, and providers are likely to see a variety of flag types, potentially leading to confusion.

Canned comments

Canned comments are standard messages programmed into the LIS that appear on patient laboratory reports for various purposes, such as providing pertinent information for result interpretation, disclaimers, or suggesting recommended follow-up.[28] Canned comments are also useful to inform a clinician when additional or reflex testing is being performed to avoid unnecessary calls to the laboratory.[28] To avoid negative impact to efficiency of the health care provider, it is pertinent to use canned comments to address frequently encountered questions and to keep the language succinct.[32] For molecular infectious disease assays, canned comments can be used for explanation of results that prompt frequent questions, such as when an organism is detected below the limit of quantification for a viral load assay. Canned comments can also be utilized to convey important information that may require further action, such as analytical sensitivity limitations when assays are highly multiplexed.[33] For example, a report comment may suggest that follow-up testing with an HSV-1 targeted PCR if M/E syndromic panel results are negative but HSV M/E is suspected.[34] When utilizing canned comments, the visibility and placement of the comment should be assessed to ensure it can be easily viewed on the laboratory reports.[28] Ideally, the comment should appear in a logical position in relation to the test result to which it applies. In both the placement and length of the comment, the efficiency of the health care provider should be considered.

Nudges

Nudging can be used postanalytically to influence behaviors, such as appropriate ordering of additional testing, while still preserving the ability of the provider to choose. In 1 study, Meeker and colleagues demonstrated that 3 different postanalytical nudging strategies (suggested alternatives, accountable justification, and peer comparison) significantly affected physician behavior toward the desired outcome, which in this case was reduction in inappropriate antibiotic prescription.[35] The 'suggested alternative' strategy presented electronic order sets of nonantibiotic treatments, the 'accountable justification' required the clinician to provide a written justification for requiring antibiotics, and 'peer comparison' provided data to the clinicians on how their rate of antibiotic prescription compared to others (with the clinicians with the lowest inappropriate prescribing rate earning the title of "top performer"). These nudging strategies can also be applied to diagnostic stewardship of costly molecular assays. For example, if a large syndromic panel is requested, a suggested alternative may be a smaller panel with clinically relevant organisms. Other electronic nudging strategies such as information transparency can be used to display cost of testing information to encourage responsible decision-making and have been shown to positively influence diagnostic stewardship.[32,36]

Clinical decision support tools

CDS tools are an important function of the EHR that utilize aggregated or inputted data to guide clinical decision-making for a specific patient.[37] CDS tools have been used for several decades in a variety of disciplines including clinical microbiology, with the notable example of antibiograms for data-driven selection of empiric antimicrobial treatment.[38,39] Most CDS tools in use today utilize expert systems, which are programmed rules from a knowledge base (which is often input from medical experts or guidelines) along with a user interface.[37] ML, a subfield of AI which uses algorithms to "learn" from large data sets, can be applied to CDS without reliance on expert systems to make interpretations, predictions, and diagnoses.[37] There have been many published studies demonstrating potential applications of ML CDS in the field of infectious disease such as prediction and early detection of sepsis, diagnosis of infection, predicting treatment responses, assisting in the choice of appropriate antibiotics or antivirals, and predicting the likelihood of antimicrobial resistance.[37] One interesting potential application is in molecular determination of antimicrobial resistance, which is typically performed by detection of gene(s) known to confer resistance by techniques such as reverse transcription PCR. However, this purely genomic approach may not accurately predict what is seen phenotypically in all organisms.[40] In 1 study, ML was trained to predict molecular markers of resistance using both genomic sequence information and gene expression data in *Pseudomonas aeruginosa* which led to high predictive values of resistance against 4 antibiotic classes.[40] While promising, more clinical studies are needed to refine the application of this technology and its use in CDS.

ML CDS tools have tremendous potential to contribute to value-based health care, but the cost and expertise to build the systems present an organizational challenge. Hurdles to implementation of ML CDS are that large data sets are required to train algorithms, so the use of ML CDS is more likely to be implemented in secondary or tertiary health care settings that have access to these larger data sets. The cost of implementation may also limit access to high socioeconomic areas. Open access databases are key to allow for implementation in primary care settings with limited patient data as well as underserved areas. For these reasons, expert systems are still valuable CDS tools and the most widely used in clinical practice.[37] Whether using expert systems or ML, the interpreted data must be presented to the health care provider and are often in the form of an alert. As mentioned previously, alerts should be used judiciously as too many can impede efficient workflow and contribute to alert fatigue.[39]

Tools in Development

Potential role of advanced artificial intelligence integration to support diagnostics stewardship

Rule-based algorithms for reflexive testing, result verification, and result commenting are examples of expert-derived AI tools in current practice. ML is an alternative AI approach that is useful for problems where expertise and knowledge are limiting factors.[41] ML algorithms come in different varieties that offer tradeoffs between accuracy, complexity, and interpretability, but the general purpose of these algorithms is to identify complex patterns in historical training data to make useful predictions for new data. There are many potential use cases for ML and AI in diagnostic stewardship, but critical gaps must be addressed to move forward, such as defining the regulatory framework for AI applications in health care.[42,43]

Prediction algorithms

Prediction algorithms identify patients at risk for negative outcomes to inform timely diagnosis and treatment. Famous examples include predictors of sepsis and acute kidney injury.[44,45] These predictions could help ensure that patients receive appropriate laboratory testing (eg, identification of patients at high risk for sepsis who may benefit from syndromic BCID panels).

Result prediction tools

Result prediction tools are trained to predict the outcome of a test based on the information available at the time of order. A confident prediction may highlight overutilization where performing the test would not be expected to provide novel information. For example, Luo and colleagues trained a predictor using laboratory data and patient demographics that could accurately predict whether a ferritin test would yield an abnormal result.[46] A potential benefit of a reliable predicted result would be a shortened turnaround time as the clinician does not have to wait for the testing process to be completed. Beyond individual results, the predictability of the results by ML has been used to screen more broadly for poor test utilization.[47,48]

Recommender tools

Recommender tools learn patterns of what tests are typically co-ordered together in a similar context to make recommendations to the ordering provider.[49–51] These tools are analogous to how algorithms from online retailers make product recommendations based on users with similar orders and browsing histories. Recommender tools could help improve laboratory utilization by identifying missed orders (underutilization) and misorders (overutilization).

Large language models

Large language models (LLMs) are massive ML models trained to learn language patterns using a huge corpus of existing texts. These models have recently advanced their capabilities as general tools for processing and generating spoken or written language. LLMs might improve utilization management by aiding in test interpretation, mining unstructured notes in the EHR, synthesizing, and summarizing external information sources, and making recommendations for test selection. A major concern with LLMs is their tendency to confidently produce inaccurate output. In 1 study, ChatGPT, a popular user interface, and LLMs, provided by OpenAI, provided incorrect responses approximately 50% of the time when prompted with laboratory medicine questions.[52] At present, clinical use cases should be limited to those where an expert reviewer can detect and correct inaccuracies.[53] Other concerns with this emerging technology include the lack of reproducibility in the output and the potential to perpetuate and amplify biases and stereotypes from the training corpus. These tools may be improved by supplemental training or context engineering using high-quality laboratory medicine–specific content and by developing domain-specific guardrail and safety systems.

SUMMARY

The electronic tools discussed earlier have the potential for measurable financial benefit and impact to patient care but often require highly sought-after information technology resources for implementation. It is imperative to utilize these tools and study their effectiveness to understand which approaches are most useful to contribute to value-based health care and diagnostic stewardship, particularly for expensive molecular microbiology tests. Benefits such as reduced ordering of molecular syndromic panels or *C difficile* PCR tests for inappropriate clinical scenarios must be quantified through relevant metrics to calculate the return on investment. Any interventions which are implemented should also be cognizant of the clinical workflow and endeavor to maximize the efficiency and user experience of the ordering physician. Finally, the application of new technology such as ML and AI for laboratory stewardship should be explored, but studies are needed to understand its accuracy and to determine how these techniques could be optimally utilized. There is also work that needs to be done to address regulatory and ethical concerns about the use of AI in laboratory medicine before it can realistically be applied.

CLINICS CARE POINTS

- Electronic tools in the electronic health record, laboratory information system, middleware, and laboratory analyzer can be intervention points for clinical decision support and laboratory stewardship.
- Preanalytical interventions, such as best practice alerts, are effective tools for optimizing laboratory test utilization, but should be used judiciously to minimize alert fatigue.
- Postanalytical interventions, such as canned comments, abnormal result flagging, and other nudging strategies, are useful to expedite result review, encourage appropriate patient management, and optimize downstream test utilization.
- Emerging technologies such as machine learning and artificial intelligence have potential to improve value-based healthcare, but significant barriers, including cost of implementation and access to data sets required for robust algorithm development, must be overcome before these tools become widely available.

DISCLOSURE

M.W. Starolis discloses that she is a full-time employee and stockholder of Quest Diagnostics. M.W. Starolis is an elected council member of the Pan American Society of Clinical Virology (PASCV), and chair of the PASCV Clinical Practice Committee. M.W. Starolis has served as an unpaid advisor to Roche and Bio-Rad. R.M. Liesman is a member of the PASCV Clinical Practice Committee. M.A. Zaydman has received speaking honoraria from Siemens and Sebia and speaking honoraria with travel support from the Association for Diagnostic and Laboratory Medicine (ADLM) and the Association of Pathology Informatics. M.A. Zaydman serves as a committee member on the ADLM Data Analytics Steering Committee. M.A. Zaydman received research support from bioMérieux. M.A. Zaydman holds provisional patents, US 20210311046 A1 and US2022/071184.

REFERENCES

1. Zhu H, Zhang H, Xu Y, et al. PCR past, present and future. Biotechniques 2020; 69(4):317–25.

2. Ramanan P, Bryson AL, Binnicker MJ, et al. Syndromic panel-based testing in clinical microbiology. Clin Microbiol Rev 2018;31(1). https://doi.org/10.1128/cmr.00024-17.
3. Gu W, Miller S, Chiu CY. Clinical metagenomic next-generation sequencing for pathogen detection. Annu Rev Pathol: Mech Dis 2018;14(1):1–20.
4. Allan GM, Lexchin J. Physician awareness of diagnostic and nondrug therapeutic costs: a systematic review. Int J Technol Assess Heal Care 2008;24(2):158–65.
5. Shanafelt TD, Dyrbye LN, Sinsky C, et al. Relationship between clerical burden and characteristics of the electronic environment with physician burnout and professional satisfaction. Mayo Clin Proc 2016;91(7):836–48.
6. Osheroff J, Teich J, Levick D, et al. Improving outcomes with clinical decision support: an implementer's guide, (HIMSS Book Series). 2nd edition. Boca Raton, FL: CRC Press/Taylor & Francis Group; 2012.
7. Ng HJH, Kansal A, Naseer JFA, et al. Optimizing best practice advisory alerts in electronic medical records with a multi-pronged strategy at a tertiary care hospital in Singapore. JAMIA Open 2023;6(3):ooad056.
8. Szymanski JJ, Qavi AJ, Laux K, et al. Once-per-visit alerts: a means to study alert compliance and reduce repeat laboratory testing. Clin Chem 2019;65(9): 1125–31.
9. Krasowski MD, Schriever A, Mathur G, et al. Use of a data warehouse at an academic medical center for clinical pathology quality improvement, education, and research. J Pathol Inform 2015;6(1):45.
10. Wolf A, Sant'Anna A, Vilhelmsson A. Using nudges to promote clinical decision making of healthcare professionals: a scoping review. Prev Med 2022;164: 107320.
11. DeSilva MB, Kodet A, Walker PF. A best practice alert for identifying hepatitis B–infected patients. Am J Trop Med Hyg 2020;103(2):884–6.
12. Luo RF, Spradley S, Banaei N. Alerting physicians during electronic order entry effectively reduces unnecessary repeat PCR testing for clostridium difficile. J Clin Microbiol 2013;51(11):3872–4.
13. Wilen CB, Monaco CL, Hoppe-Bauer J, et al. Criteria for reducing unnecessary testing for herpes simplex virus, varicella-zoster virus, cytomegalovirus, and enterovirus in cerebrospinal fluid samples from adults. J Clin Microbiol 2015; 53(3):887–95.
14. Lang T. Minimum retesting intervals in practice: 10 years experience. Clin Chem Lab Med 2021;59(1):39–50.
15. Mandelia Y, Procop GW, Richter SS, et al. Optimal timing of repeat multiplex molecular testing for respiratory viruses. J Clin Microbiol 2020;58(2). https://doi.org/10.1128/jcm.01203-19.
16. Hitchcock MM, Gomez CA, Banaei N. Low yield of filmarray gi panel in hospitalized patients with diarrhea: an opportunity for diagnostic stewardship intervention. J Clin Microbiol 2018;56(3). https://doi.org/10.1128/jcm.01558-17.
17. Park S, Hitchcock MM, Gomez CA, et al. Is follow-up testing with the filmarray gastrointestinal multiplex PCR panel necessary? J Clin Microbiol 2017;55(4): 1154–61.
18. Kraft CS, Parrott JS, Cornish NE, et al. A laboratory medicine best practices systematic review and meta-analysis of nucleic acid amplification tests (NAATs) and algorithms including NAATs for the diagnosis of clostridioides (Clostridium) difficile in adults. Clin Microbiol Rev 2019;32(3):000322–418.

19. Feldman LS, Shihab HM, Thiemann D, et al. Impact of providing fee data on laboratory test ordering: a controlled clinical trial. JAMA Intern Med 2013;173(10):903–8.
20. Escovedo C, Bell D, Cheng E, et al. Noninterruptive clinical decision support decreases ordering of respiratory viral panels during influenza season. Appl Clin Inform 2020;11(02):315–22.
21. Howard-Anderson JR, Sexton ME, Robichaux C, et al. The impact of an electronic medical record nudge on reducing testing for hospital-onset Clostridioides difficile infection. Infect Control Hosp Epidemiol 2020;41(4):411–7.
22. Hamilton R, Pandora TR, Parsonnet J, et al. Clinical decision support trees can help optimize utilization of anaplasma phagocytophilum nucleic acid amplification testing. J Clin Microbiol 2021;59(9):007911–21.
23. Madden GR, Mesner IG, Cox HL, et al. Reduced clostridium difficile tests and laboratory-identified events with a computerized clinical decision support tool and financial incentive. Infect Control Hosp Epidemiol 2018;39(6):737–40.
24. Chen H, Butler E, Guo Y, et al. Facilitation or hindrance: physicians' perception on best practice alerts (BPA) usage in an electronic health record system. Heal Commun 2019;34(9):942–8.
25. Procop GW, Keating C, Stagno P, et al. Reducing duplicate testinga comparison of two clinical decision support tools. Am J Clin Pathol 2015;143(5):623–6.
26. Powers EM, Shiffman RN, Melnick ER, et al. Efficacy and unintended consequences of hard-stop alerts in electronic health record systems: a systematic review. J Am Méd Inform Assoc 2018;25(11):1556–66.
27. Broadhurst MJ, Dujari S, Budvytiene I, et al. Utilization, yield, and accuracy of the filmarray meningitis/encephalitis panel with diagnostic stewardship and testing algorithm. J Clin Microbiol 2020;58(9). https://doi.org/10.1128/jcm.00311-20.
28. Ruff HM, Poonawala H, Sebastian C, et al. Canned comments in the hospital laboratory information system can decrease microbiology requests. Am J Clin Pathol 2021;156(6):1155–61.
29. Force UPST, Owens DK, Davidson KW, et al. Screening for hepatitis c virus infection in adolescents and adults. JAMA 2020;323(10):970–5.
30. Harrison J. OIG Compliance Guidelines Federal Register. Published online 1998. Available at: https://oig.hhs.gov/documents/compliance-guidance/806/cpglab.pdf. Accessed September 29, 2023.
31. Lum G. Critical limits (alert values) for physician notification: universal or medical center specific limits? Ann Clin Lab Sci 1998;28(5):261–71.
32. Sedrak MS, Myers JS, Small DS, et al. Effect of a price transparency intervention in the electronic health record on clinician ordering of inpatient laboratory tests: the price randomized clinical trial. JAMA Intern Med 2017;177(7):939.
33. Trujillo-Gómez J, Tsokani S, Arango-Ferreira C, et al. Biofire filmarray meningitis/encephalitis panel for the aetiological diagnosis of central nervous system infections: a systematic review and diagnostic test accuracy meta-analysis. eClinicalMedicine 2022;44:101275.
34. Gaensbauer J, Fernholz E, Hiskey L, et al. Comparison of two assays to diagnose herpes simplex virus in patients with central nervous system infections. J Clin Virol 2023;166:105528.
35. Meeker D, Linder JA, Fox CR, et al. Effect of behavioral interventions on inappropriate antibiotic prescribing among primary care practices: a randomized clinical trial. JAMA 2016;315(6):562–70.

36. Santos RP, Deutschendorf C, Vido HG, et al. Antimicrobial stewardship: the influence of behavioral nudging on renal-function–based appropriateness of dosing. Infect Control Hosp Epidemiol 2020;41(9):1077–9.
37. Peiffer-Smadja N, Rawson TM, Ahmad R, et al. Machine learning for clinical decision support in infectious diseases: a narrative review of current applications. Clin Microbiol Infect 2020;26(5):584–95.
38. Rhoads DD, Sintchenko V, Rauch CA, et al. Clinical microbiology informatics. Clin Microbiol Rev 2014;27(4):1025–47.
39. Mills S. Electronic health records and use of clinical decision support. Crit Care Nurs Clin North Am 2019;31(2):125–31.
40. Khaledi A, Weimann A, Schniederjans M, et al. Predicting antimicrobial resistance in Pseudomonas aeruginosa with machine learning-enabled molecular diagnostics. EMBO Mol Med 2020;12(3):e10264.
41. Master SR, Badrick TC, Bietenbeck A, et al. Machine learning in laboratory medicine: recommendations of the IFCC working group. Clin Chem 2023;69(7):690–8.
42. Rabbani N, Kim GYE, Suarez CJ, et al. Applications of machine learning in routine laboratory medicine: current state and future directions. Clin Biochem 2022; 103:1–7.
43. Durant TJS, MD. Machine Learning and Laboratory Medicine: Now and the Road Ahead. Available at: https://www.aacc.org/cln/articles/2019/march/machine-learning-and-laboratory-medicine-now-and-the-road-ahead. Accessed September 29, 2023.
44. Fleuren LM, Klausch TLT, Zwager CL, et al. Machine learning for the prediction of sepsis: a systematic review and meta-analysis of diagnostic test accuracy. Intensiv Care Med 2020;46(3):383–400.
45. Tomašev N, Glorot X, Rae JW, et al. A clinically applicable approach to continuous prediction of future acute kidney injury. Nature 2019;572(7767):116–9.
46. Luo Y, Szolovits P, Dighe AS, et al. Using machine learning to predict laboratory test results. Am J Clin Pathol 2016;145(6):778–88.
47. Lidbury BA, Richardson AM, Badrick T. Assessment of machine-learning techniques on large pathology data sets to address assay redundancy in routine liver function test profiles. Diagnosis 2015;2(1):41–51.
48. Xu S, Hom J, Balasubramanian S, et al. Prevalence and predictability of low-yield inpatient laboratory diagnostic tests. JAMA Netw Open 2019;2(9):e1910967.
49. Kumar A, Aikens RC, Hom J, et al. OrderRex clinical user testing: a randomized trial of recommender system decision support on simulated cases. J Am Méd Inform Assoc 2020;27(12):ocaa190.
50. Chen JH, Goldstein MK, Asch SM, et al. Predicting inpatient clinical order patterns with probabilistic topic models vs conventional order sets. J Am Méd Inform Assoc 2017;24(3):472–80.
51. Islam MM, Yang HC, Poly TN, et al. Development of an artificial intelligence–based automated recommendation system for clinical laboratory tests: retrospective analysis of the national health insurance database. JMIR Méd Inform 2020; 8(11):e24163.
52. Munoz-Zuluaga C, Zhao Z, Wang F, et al. Assessing the accuracy and clinical utility of ChatGPT in laboratory medicine. Clin Chem 2023;69(8):939–40.
53. Snyder C, Zaydman MA, Chong T, et al. Generative artificial intelligence: more of the same or off the control chart? Clin Chem 2023;69(10):1101–6.

Present and Future Non-Culture-Based Diagnostics: Stewardship Potentials and Considerations

Arryn Crancy, PhD[a], Steve Miller, MD, PhD[b,*]

KEYWORDS

• Molecular microbiology • Diagnostic stewardship • Medical microbiologist
• Test implementation

KEY POINTS

- Molecular methods are replacing organism culture with improvements in test performance, but limitations remain.
- Molecular methods may be targeted or broad-based for organism detection and characterization.
- Clinical microbiologists must consider the clinical impacts and resource utilization when determining which assays to perform in their laboratory.
- Communication and education about increasingly complex results and laboratory network coordination are essential in microbiology.
- Further developments in test automation and new analysis techniques will enhance the laboratory diagnostic ability.

INTRODUCTION

Diagnostics for infectious diseases are evolving, creating a complicated landscape of testing options. This is redefining the clinical microbiology laboratory and each laboratory must assess emerging methodologies and new technologies to determine what testing best suits the needs of their patient populations and fit the infrastructure and resources in the laboratory. The goal of the publication is to provide an overview of the molecular diagnostic landscape for infectious disease diagnostics and outline considerations during molecular testing implementation. For simplicity, molecular testing is described as target-based testing referring to those tests with molecular

[a] Center for Infectious Disease Diagnostics and Research, Diagnostic Medicine Institute, Geisinger Health System, 100 North Academy Avenue, Danville, PA 17822, USA; [b] Delve Bio, Inc. and Department of Laboratory Medicine, University of California San Francisco, 953 Indiana Street, San Francisco, CA 94107, USA
* Corresponding author.
E-mail address: steve.miller@delve.bio

Clin Lab Med 44 (2024) 109–122
https://doi.org/10.1016/j.cll.2023.10.003

detection using defined targets and broad-based testing referring to those tests relying on next-generation sequencing (NGS) methodologies.

One size does not fit all laboratories and the role of the medical microbiologist is to liaise with others to implement changes to diagnostic testing as new testing options come available. As non-culture-based diagnostics grow and new testing methodologies and algorithms emerge, the role of the medical microbiologist will be vital in implementing and maintaining diagnostic testing for infectious diseases.

TRANSITION TO MOLECULAR-BASED DIAGNOSTICS

Culture-based diagnostics have been the mainstay diagnostic tool in the clinical microbiology laboratory due to numerous advantages, including low cost and ability to provide antimicrobial susceptibility testing (AST) for the specific patient's isolate (**Table 1**).[1] However, culture-based diagnostics do not capture all pathogens, are labor-intensive to perform, and require an extensive incubation time (days to weeks/months) and a plethora of specialized media to allow for microbe growth.

Non-culture-based diagnostics, especially molecular diagnostics, are proving their diagnostic value, and clinical microbiology is moving toward further adoption of molecular techniques (see **Table 1**).[2] The ability to automate molecular diagnostic testing, the typically improved sensitivity, and the reduced time to pathogen detection in comparison to culture are some of the primary factors that favor adoption of molecular diagnostics.

Table 1
Advantages and disadvantages of culture versus molecular assays for clinical microbiology

Technique	Advantages	Disadvantages
Culture	• Often the gold standard test • Isolate recovery demonstrates viability • Isolates enable antibiotic susceptibility testing • Low cost and less reliance on specialized equipment	• Not all pathogens are recoverable by culture • Pathogens need to remain viable after collection • Long turnaround times (days to weeks/months) • Labor intensive to perform • Highly technical to train diagnostic techniques • Assay variation due to technologist level reporting • Labor force is dwindling • Requires a plethora of specialized media
Molecular	• Improved sensitivity over culture • Does not require the pathogen to be viable • Many commercial assays • Sample to answer format promotes adoption • Detects multiple pathogens in a single test • Reduces turnaround time • Automatable workflow • Quantitative testing, informing on the abundance • Able to create own assays	• Many options with varying equipment/staff requirements • Isolate not be available for antibiotic susceptibility testing • Should be coordinated with diagnostic stewardship • Risk of false positives • Requires dedicated workflow • Targeted approaches require suspected pathogen list • Sample to answer formats generates significant waste • Does not inform on the viability of the pathogen • Reimbursement may be variable

This transition in diagnostics will better support the clinical microbiology laboratory as laboratories deal with a dwindling workforce that requires extensive specialized training.[3]

The rapid increase in molecular diagnostics has created a mosaic of molecular testing options (**Table 2**). These testing options can be organized by the type of molecular information collected for the assay. Target-based molecular testing are assays that detect a defined list of pathogens or antibiotic resistance (AMR) genes and can be divided into ones where only a single pathogen or multiple pathogens (syndromic/multiplexed) are detected. Broad-based molecular testing are assays that interrogate all genetic information in the sample and can be divided into whole-genome sequencing (WGS) and metagenomics applications.

As part of the advancement in molecular diagnostics, the workflow requirements for molecular testing have been greatly simplified by many commercial manufacturers, enabling adoption of molecular diagnostics outside a traditional molecular laboratory, including waived and over-the-counter testing in some cases.[4,5] As well, the lowered cost of NGS has created opportunities to explore applications for agnostic pathogen detection (metagenomics) and WGS as diagnostic tools in the clinical microbiology laboratory.[6]

DECISION POINTS FOR IMPLEMENTING MOLECULAR TESTING

As the technology and clinical knowledge base for non-culture-based diagnostics have matured, these assays have become increasingly incorporated into routine microbiology diagnostic laboratories.[7] The medical microbiologist plays a key role in determining which assays will be offered to providers within their health care organization, and must understand the scientific basis, assess the technological methods and performance characteristics, and determine the clinical utility of these assays when applied to the intended patient population. They must also incorporate logistical, workflow, and cost considerations when selecting among available test methods to achieve efficient and clinically meaningful results for their laboratories.

Although the transition from culture to molecular test methods can improve diagnostic performance, care must be taken to vet the underlying science and technological development and understand the longevity of current assays. With available methods moving from single amplicon to multiplex panels to unbiased organism detection, there is a need to continuously adapt to newer testing platforms while still maintaining continuity to allow for effective patient care. The medical microbiologist must educate other providers about how changes to test methods impact their diagnostic performance and how this affects clinical decision-making.

Quality Considerations

A primary role for the medical microbiologist is to ensure that the test results are accurate and reliably performed in a quality operating environment. The benefits and limitations of molecular test methods compared with culture need to be carefully considered along with the factors that may cause false-positive or false-negative results. In many cases, molecular organism detection is more sensitive than culture, especially for fastidious species. This increased sensitivity is often a benefit but can return positive results in scenarios where the clinical relevance is questionable, such as detection of dead organisms. False-positive results can occur when amplification targets are not specific for the pathogen, such as shared genetic regions between rhinovirus and enteroviruses for respiratory virus panels[8] or contamination with intranasal influenza vaccine material.[9] False-negative results can occur due to assay failure or when the target of interest is not present for some pathogenic strains, such as the loss of the cryptic plasmid target

Table 2
Comparison of molecular assay types for clinical microbiology

Molecular Category	Assay Type	Assay Examples	Pros	Cons
Targeted Molecular	Single pathogen	Sputum: *M tuberculosis,* Stool: *C difficile*, Blood: HIV, HCV, HBV, VZV, HSV, Nasal: MSSA/MRSA	• Some clinical scenarios warrant single pathogen testing • Convenient formats (sample to answer) for implementation in the clinical laboratory, or in some cases waived testing and over-the-counter testing	• Each test requires its own validation and investment in the testing platform
	Syndromic/ multiplexed panels	Sexually transmitted infections, upper respiratory viral pathogens, tick borne illnesses, community-acquired meningitis, lower respiratory infections, bone and joint infections, gastrointestinal infections, bloodstream infections	• Some clinical scenarios have a broad differential warranting testing of multiple pathogens • Providing one test with clinically related pathogens simplifies testing	• Individual panels may have some targets with diagnostic issues requiring reflex testing • May result in an overreliance on syndromic testing • Can be challenging to choose the appropriate panel size to cover different patient populations
Broad Molecular	WGS	Variant typing, epidemiologic investigations, AMR prediction	• Pandemic preparedness to identify novel pathogens of unknown origin • Provides detailed genetic information of a single organism	• Generally, an assay will be research use only • Technology barrier to mainstream adoption • Requires extensive validation • Genotypic AMR detection may not correlate with phenotypic results
	Metagenomics (targeted and unbiased)	Pathogen detection from body fluids and tissues	• Pandemic preparedness to identify novel pathogens of unknown origin • Agnostic pathogen detection in a single test direct from specimen	• Relatively few laboratories offer clinical metagenomic testing • Technology barrier to mainstream adoption • Requires extensive validation to report results clinically • Antibiotic resistance information is provided at the resistome level • Resistome reporting for AMR detected may not link to the exact pathogen/infectious processes

Abbreviations: HBV, Hepatitis B Virus; HCV, Hepatitis C Virus; HIV, Human Immunodeficiency Virus; HSV, Herpes Simplex Virus; MRSA, Methicillin-Resistant Staph-

that was used for detection of *Chlamydia trachomatis*.[10] Molecular resistance testing is another example where multiple mechanisms may occur that limit the detection range, such as when methicillin-resistant *Staphylococcus aureus* is due to the mecC gene rather than the more common mecA gene.[11] Over time, improvements in assay design can overcome these limitations, but there remains a need for continued surveillance and suspicion for novel pathogen emergence that might require assay refinement.

Patient Impacts

A major consideration for implementation of a new molecular test will be the potential for patient benefit via improved diagnostic efficacy. This should be assessed in a metric-driven manner, reviewing the diagnostic yield and turnaround time along with the impact on patient management. Molecular detection of viruses via polymerase chain reaction (PCR) or other amplification methods has largely supplanted traditional viral culture in most clinical laboratories, because the increase in sensitivity and decrease in turnaround time has a clear benefit to patient care.[12] The decision to switch to molecular detection for toxigenic *Clostridioides difficile* required more investigation and education on how to approach patients with suspected *C difficile*-associated diarrhea. The prior approach of cell culture cytotoxicity assay took several days to yield a result but was more sensitive than toxin antigen detection assays. PCR clearly demonstrated more rapid detection for *C difficile* organism and toxin genes but would also identify patients as positive who were simply colonized with toxigenic *C difficile*.[13] In this case, PCR detection of the toxin gene may be overly sensitive for accurate diagnosis, and further testing using a less sensitive antigen assay may be considered to distinguish true infection from likely colonization. As laboratories have adopted molecular testing for *C difficile*, considerable effort has been needed steward testing only when appropriate and to educate providers about the meaning of positive molecular toxin detection versus antigen detection to guide the use of specific *C difficile* therapy.[14]

Logistics and Cost

As molecular testing advances for infectious diseases, the practical side of operating and expenses in the laboratory must be accounted for. There are now a variety of testing platforms to choose from, each with a different test menu, mechanism, and performance characteristics. Laboratories often will consolidate their test menu on certain instruments due to physical space constraints and the cost of maintaining multiple instrument types. Some of these can be used for laboratory developed testing procedures (LDPs), which can take significant resources to develop and validate for clinical use. The medical microbiologist must balance the need to offer a variety of test methods with the resources required to maintain each of these and consider whether the turnaround time requires in-house versus reference testing. As more molecular testing systems with expanded test menus are developed, there are increasing numbers of options for microbiology laboratories to expand their test offerings to meet provider demands. Reimbursement rates and the size of molecular test panels are also considered when evaluating the economic impact to the laboratory and health care organization.

Resource Considerations

The medical microbiologist must be cognizant of the laboratory resources available to support the variety of methodologies and technologies needed to provide test results for patient care. The laboratory space configuration and staffing will partially determine what level of service can be provided, with centralized laboratories offering higher throughput and disseminated laboratories offering more rapid turnaround time but requiring higher staffing levels, especially if instruments are placed in multiple locations. Implementation of new assays offers opportunities for education and stewardship program development to ensure that laboratory resources are used efficiently and tests are ordered on the appropriate patient care population. Stewardship efforts are best done in collaboration with other departments including infection control, infectious disease, and individual units. Protocols guiding the ordering or reflex testing for more expensive molecular tests can help maximize their utility, such as decision criteria, for which patients will benefit from a rapid multiplex PCR panel identification of positive blood cultures.[15] More complex assays such as metagenomic pathogen detection may benefit from infectious disease physician consult services, so that the decision on appropriate testing can be applied on an individual case basis.[16] The medical microbiologist plays a key role to coordinate guideline development and ensure that these protocols serve the needs of various clinical departments.

MOLECULAR TEST USE CASES

There are two overall requirements for replacing culture-based diagnostics: pathogen identification and AST. Although not all pathogens require AST to provide targeted antibiotic therapy to the patient, those pathogens recovered by culture-based diagnostics typically do and molecular diagnostics must be developed for AMR prediction before culture can be fully replaced. Molecular diagnostics for pathogen identification have been extensively developed (see **Table 2**) and little barriers for adoption exist. However, the ability of molecular diagnostics to reliably predict AMR detection is currently limited.[17] Assays are available for the detection of discrete AMR genes for hospital-acquired infections (mecA gene in *S aureus*, vanA/B gene in *Enterococcus faecalis* and *E faecium*, and klebsiella pneumoniae carbapenemase (KPC), imipenemase (IMP), New Delhi Metallo-beta-lactamase (NDM), verona integron-encoded metallo-beta-lactamase (VIM) in Gram-negative bacteria) or well-characterized single-nucleotide polymorphisms (SNPs) known to confer AMR. *Mycobacterium* is particularly suited for SNP-based AMR prediction. Many genes are well characterized (katG, rpoB, gyrA/B, and others) in *M tuberculosis* which predict resistance to a combination of antibiotics used to treat tuberculosis (Rifampin, Isoniazid, Pyrazinamide, and Ethambutol) RIPE therapy[18] and the rrl gene for clarithromycin and rrs gene for amikacin in non-tuberculate mycobacteria.[19] Laboratories have the opportunity to develop LDPs for AMR prediction. Although AMR prediction is lagging in comparison to pathogen identification, many opportunities for molecular diagnostics exist where AST is either not required or molecular prediction is sufficient.

Uses for Target-Based Molecular Methods: Single Pathogen

The most common molecular assays in the clinical microbiology laboratory are target-based. Single pathogen targeted assays tend to be used for surveillance purposes and decisions during hospital admissions (see **Table 2**). For example, direct from sputum molecular detection is used to rule out *M tuberculosis* and assessing nasal swabs for MRSA carriage before surgery guides prophylaxis.[20] The detection of *C difficile* will guide infection prevention practices in the patient's room[21] and the respiratory viral status can be assessed quickly to prevent antibiotic overuse.[22]

Uses for Target-Based Molecular Methods: Syndromic/Multiplexed Panels

Syndromic/multiplexed panels provide testing options for when clinical scenarios possess broad differentials with overlapping symptoms to quickly identify the infectious agents and generally require coordination with diagnostic stewardship to fully reap the benefits.[23,24] With the exception of syndromic panels for bloodstream infections, syndromic panels focus on opportunities that do not require AST. For example, syndromic testing for respiratory infections has centered on viral pathogens and fastidious bacteria that do not grow in culture.[25] Infectious causes of gastrointestinal illnesses have overlapping symptoms, can be caused by a number of bacterial, viral, and parasite pathogens, are generally self-resolving and little AST is required. Similarly, syndromic panels exist for the most common bacterial, fungal, and viral causes of community-acquired meningitis with only the patients testing positive for a bacterial or fungal pathogen requiring phenotypic AST testing.[26] Syndromic panels for bloodstream infections are used on positive blood cultures as an adjuvant to culture to provide early identification of the pathogen and typically include detection of the discrete AMR genes for hospital-acquired infections like mecA, vanA, KPC, IMP, NDM, and VIM.[27]

Uses for Broad-Based Molecular Methods: Metagenomics

Clinical use of broad-based molecular applications is increasing, but testing is usually sequestered to academic medical centers, public health, and reference laboratories due to the requirement for specialized equipment and training. Metagenomics is gaining favor for its ability to agnostically assess pathogens directly from a specimen.[28,29] This is of particular value for specimen types that are typically sterile. Metagenomic techniques are classed as targeted or unbiased. Targeted metagenomics relies on primers to amplify genes of interests for detection. The 16S and internal transcribed spacer (ITS) sequences are popular for bacterial and fungal identification, respectively. Unbiased metagenomics relies on shotgun sequencing to interrogate the specimen with bioinformatic analysis to identify microbial sequences present in the sample.

Uses for Broad-Based Molecular Methods: Whole-Genome Sequencing

WGS is used for isolate characterization, interrogating the genetic information of a particular pathogen in detail to determine the exact strain and genetic determinants. This level of resolution can be used in real-time monitoring of strain variants coupled with infection prevention interventions to curb nosocomial transmissions.[30] WGS also has value in AMR predictions providing the exact isolate for analysis without the contribution of other microorganisms in the specimen. As well, investment in NGS diagnostics enables the laboratory to have the functionality to participate in research aspects required to further develop diagnostics for AMR prediction.[31]

LABORATORY NETWORK COORDINATION IN MICROBIOLOGY

The global COVID-19 outbreak clearly demonstrated the importance of coordination among laboratories to ensure availability of sufficient diagnostic testing and microbiologic surveillance. Limited resources required the allocation of sample collection and testing supplies based on need and capacity considerations, and sequencing programs had to be rapidly expanded to perform SARS-CoV-2 genomic sequencing to track epidemiologic trends in viral strain transmission and identify novel variants.[32] The medical microbiologist plays a key role to coordinate testing among laboratories offering different types of assays and services. Individual clinical microbiology laboratories interact with clinical reference, public health, and research laboratories in a variety of situations to complete diagnostic workups and contribute to disease surveillance and new test development activities (**Fig. 1**).

Clinical Reference Laboratories

The primary role of the clinical microbiology laboratory is to perform diagnostic testing to inform patient care decisions within a health care organization. As the spectrum of

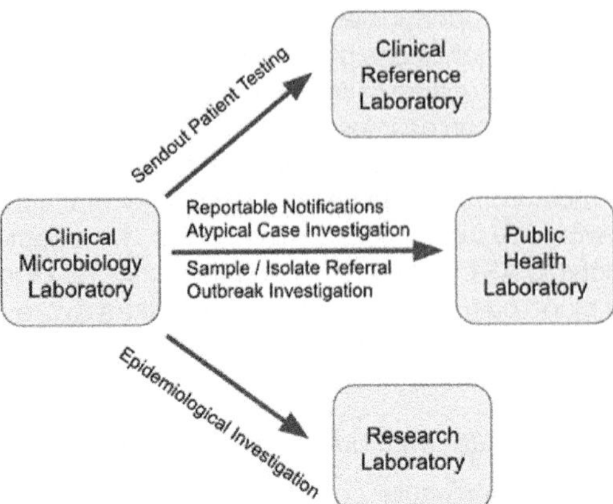

Fig. 1. Laboratory network coordination. Interaction of the clinical microbiology laboratory with clinical reference, public health and research laboratories in support of patient care, and infectious disease surveillance activities.

diagnostic assays expands, there are many more tests available than can be performed within an individual laboratory. The rapid expansion of molecular diagnostic assays is a significant contributor to the proliferation of potential test methods, and each laboratory must make decisions about which tests to perform in-house and which to send out to reference laboratories. The medical microbiologist must assess which test methods to offer based on available resources, staffing, cost, and need for rapid turnaround time for patient care. Lower volume tests and those requiring specialized training or equipment, including many molecular diagnostic methods, are typically only available as sendout tests to reference laboratories, and their use may be restricted by institutional policy based on cost and patient care considerations.

Public Health Laboratories

Beyond direct patient care testing, an often overlooked role of the clinical microbiology laboratory is to support local and national public health programs. Because clinical microbiology laboratories are often the first sites to receive samples from patients with suspected infections, they serve as sentinel laboratories within the public health system.[33] These laboratories are mandated to report cases that meet criteria for laboratory-notifiable conditions as defined by local public health authorities and may also be required to forward certain types of patient samples for further analysis. The goal of these policies is to identify new cases and outbreaks of infectious disease so that appropriate public health interventions can be taken to limit spread in the population. Microbial strain typing and identification of toxigenic strains are useful tools to investigate potential infectious disease outbreaks and guide the public health response.

The expansion of non-culture-based methods to diagnose infections has affected public health investigations and required changes to the methods used for these investigations. Culture methods would typically provide a microbial isolate that can be stored, shipped, and expanded for further analysis such as strain typing, resistance testing, and serotyping. Without a cultured isolate, only primary patient samples are available for these types of tests, and the sample volumes may be too small to allow for multiple assays to be performed. Molecular panels for direct detection of stool pathogens have improved patient diagnosis due to improved sensitivity and turnaround time in the clinical laboratory,[34] but determining the bacterial strain type is more difficult directly from the stool sample. Public health laboratories have to attempt to obtain and perform culture or molecular-based typing methods from patient stool samples.[35] Culture-independent target amplification or metagenomic sequencing assays can be used to characterize the pathogens present in these samples and inform infection rates and expansion in the population.

Public health laboratories may offer clinically validated assays meeting Clinical Laboratory Improvements Act standards so that the results can be used for patient care decisions as part of the medical record. These specialized assays can be used to identify toxigenic or virulent bacterial strains, identify atypical isolates via genomic sequencing, or detect vector-borne viruses that are monitored for public health programs. Several laboratories that are part of the Centers for Disease Control network have been working to enable clinical use for their assays. Although these tests may have prolonged turnaround times, they are a significant resource for advanced molecular diagnostics that may not be available through reference laboratories.

Research Laboratories

Research laboratories may use patient samples in their studies with appropriate institutional research board approval. These studies often use de-identified patient samples to minimize any risk of release of private health information and may include information from clinical sample test results or other data abstracted from the patient chart. These studies often investigate infectious disease epidemiology, pathogenicity, or develop new methods that can be applied to diagnostic testing. Results from these studies are not reported to individual patients or intended to be used for patient care decisions.

In some cases, there is a need to further characterize patient samples using methods that are available only in research laboratories. These can involve strain typing from patient samples where there is a suspected outbreak within a hospital or other health care setting. In these cases, an investigation may be performed by the institutional infection control department to determine whether pathogen transmission within the health care environment is taking place, and the results can inform measures to prevent further transmission. Results from these studies are not used for individual patient care decisions but are incorporated into the institutional quality assurance program to guide infection control measures. These can include removal of medical devices such as contaminated endoscopes from patient use[36] or isolation and infection precaution measures used in particular hospital units.[37] Metagenomic sequencing methods to compare pathogen genomes have been used to rule out transmission in suspected outbreaks,[38] which can translate to significant cost savings in the hospital setting.

FUTURE DIRECTIONS

The adaptation of non-culture-based diagnostic methods to clinical microbiology will continue to rapidly advance, improving assay performance for organism detection. These tests will increasingly include the ability to identify molecular markers of diagnostic value such as antimicrobial resistance genes and perform strain typing. These assays will have applications for microbial isolate characterization and direct specimen analysis and provide more complex results that will need to be properly communicated to treating clinicians. This information will also provide better understanding of pathogen transmission dynamics for public health monitoring and more rapidly detect novel agents with pandemic potential. The medical microbiologist will continue to have a significant role in the selection of appropriate testing methods for their patient population and interpretation of molecular markers relevant to infectious disease.

Automation

With the dwindling workforce of trained medical laboratory scientists (MLS) and ever-expanding demand for higher volume and more diverse testing methods, the automation of molecular diagnostics is now a requirement for survival for many clinical microbiology laboratories. There are currently a variety of sample-to-answer molecular test platforms with microbiology test menus available. Even traditional culture methods are becoming automated with systems that can perform media inoculation, incubation, and culture reading in an automated fashion. One can imagine a future MLS spending much of their time reviewing and verifying results at their computer rather than directly handling culture plates or reading cultures. On the hospital systems level, economic pressures will continue to lead to consolidation of centralized microbiology laboratories along with the shift to near patient and point-of-care testing where rapid results can improve patient management. The microbiology laboratory infrastructure will have to adapt to this changing reality and provide guidance to ensure that proper testing procedures are performed in non-laboratory settings to achieve quality patient care.

Host Analysis

Methods to interrogate the human immunologic response to infections are being rapidly developed, and we can expect some of these to enter mainstream diagnostic testing in the near future. More traditional immunologic assays such as serology and flow cytometry will be supplemented with genetic analysis tools to provide insight into the patient response to the pathogenic agent. Sequencing-based tests such as metagenomic pathogen detection assays are immediately applicable for this approach, because most of the data are actually derived from the host and can be mined for patterns or markers of clinical significance.[39] Incorporation of host-derived markers for diagnosis or prognosis of infection will help to stratify patients for treatment based on their individual risk of disease progression, and expertise in microbiology will be needed to put these results into the clinical context.

Databases and Computational Infrastructure

As molecular testing grows for clinical microbiology, the methods to store and process data at the institutional level need to be considered. In particular, NGS assays generate large amounts of data and require complex bioinformatic processing pipelines needing substantial computational power and data storage capacity. The expertise needed for this type of testing is often outside the traditional clinical laboratory domain, and new support mechanisms are required to meet the computational needs while maintaining regulatory, privacy, and quality standards.

Analysis and interpretation of high-throughput sequencing data also requires large and curated databases to ensure both sensitivity (complete coverage of relevant genetic markers for pathogen/strain/host marker detection) and specificity (markers have been vetted to be properly associated with the listed organism type) for these assays. The largest publicly accessible databases such as Genbank contain many errors and misannotations, whereas highly curated databases such as Food and Drug Administration (FDA)-Argos remain limited in scope.[40] Microbiologists interpreting these assays will need to understand the databases used and their limitations when applying these results to patient care.

Decision Support and Data Science

The increased amount and complexity of molecular data being generated for diagnostic use holds substantial promise in generating individualized precision medicine for patient care decisions but also risks misinterpretation and loss of important results due to information overload. WGS for microbial organisms is now readily achievable on a routine basis, but systems to analyze these data and put it into actionable form are still being developed.[41] Future medical microbiologists will need to evaluate clinical decision support software that will distill large amounts of data into understandable and meaningful reports. These systems may include patient clinical data to help provide a comprehensive snapshot with increased diagnostic ability. Epidemiologic surveillance methods will also become more sophisticated to incorporate genomic data to track institutional and community outbreaks. Medical microbiologists will have many opportunities to help develop and guide implementation of these systems at their own institutions.

SUMMARY

The diagnostics microbiology laboratory is rapidly evolving with greater demand for more detailed clinically actionable information about pathogenic microbes in a faster time frame. The expansion of molecular methods for organism detection and characterization is poised to change the focus of laboratories from culture-based to genomic-based analysis, and the medical microbiologist will have to guide this transition to ensure that testing supports optimal patient care decisions at their organizations. The shift from targeted pathogen assays to multiplex syndromic-based panels and hypothesis-free unbiased metagenomic analysis will require substantial education and development of best practice guidelines supported by clinical evidence to realize the benefits for patient care.

CLINICS CARE POINTS

- A multitude of technologies are available for molecular infectious disease testing with varying functionality and resource needs to fit testing option needs in the research, public health and clinical laboratories.
- Molecular diagnostics for infectious diseases offer rapid and accurate identification of microbial pathogens, leading to timely treatment decisions when combined with stewardship.
- Next-generation sequencing in microbiology can guide personalized treatment options by identifying specific microbial pathogens and can assist in tracing the source of infections during outbreaks, allowing for containment and preventive measures.

DISCLOSURE

A Craney consulting for BugSeq Inc. S Miller employed by and stock options at Delve Bio Inc and holds multiple patents related to metagenomic sequencing for infectious disease.

REFERENCES

1. Bailey A, Ledeboer N, Burnham C. Clinical microbiology is growing up: the total laboratory automation revolution. Clin Chem 2019;65(5):634–43.

2. Lewinski MA, Alby K, Babady NE, et al. Exploring the utility of multiplex infectious disease panel testing for diagnosis of infection in different body sites: a joint report of the association for molecular pathology, American society for microbiology, infectious diseases society of America, and pan American society for clinical virology. J Mol Diagn 2023;S1525-1578(23):00209X.
3. Doern CD, Miller MB, Alby K, et al, American Society for Microbiology ASM Clinical and Public Health Microbiology Committee and the ASM Corporate Council. American society for microbiology (ASM) clinical and public health microbiology committee and the ASM corporate council. proceedings of the clinical microbiology open 2018 and 2019 - a discussion about emerging trends, challenges, and the future of clinical microbiology. J Clin Microbiol 2022;60(7):e0009222.
4. Bălan AM, Bodolea C, Trancă SD, et al. Trends in molecular diagnosis of nosocomial pneumonia classic PCR vs. point-of-care PCR: a narrative review. Healthcare (Basel) 2023;11(9):1345.
5. Babady NE. The FilmArray® respiratory panel: an automated, broadly multiplexed molecular test for the rapid and accurate detection of respiratory pathogens. Expert Rev Mol Diagn 2013;13(8):779–88.
6. Forbes JD, Knox NC, Ronholm J, et al. Metagenomics: the next culture-independent game changer. Front Microbiol 2017;8:1069.
7. Liu Q, Jin X, Cheng J, et al. Advances in the application of molecular diagnostic techniques for the detection of infectious disease pathogens (Review). Mol Med Rep 2023;27:104.
8. Andres C, Piñana M, Vila J, et al. The high genetic similarity between rhinoviruses and enteroviruses remains as a pitfall for molecular diagnostic tools: a three-year overview. Infect Genet Evol 2019;75:103996.
9. Bennett S, MacLean AR, Reynolds A, et al. False positive influenza A and B detections in clinical samples due to contamination with live attenuated influenza vaccine. J Med Microbiol 2015;64:466–8.
10. Stothard DR, Williams JA, Van Der Pol B, et al. Identification of a Chlamydia trachomatis serovar E urogenital isolate which lacks the cryptic plasmid. Infect Immun 1998;66:6010–3.
11. McClure JA, Conly JM, Obasuyi O, et al. A novel assay for detection of methicillin-resistant *Staphylococcus aureus* directly from clinical samples. Front Microbiol 2020;11:1295.
12. Capraro GA. Replacement of culture with molecular testing for diagnosis infectious diseases. Clin Lab Med 2022;42:547–55.
13. Polage CR, Gyorke CE, Kennedy MA, et al. Overdiagnosis of clostridium difficile infection in the molecular test era. JAMA Intern Med 2015;175:1792–801.
14. Solanky D, Juang DK, Johns ST, et al. Using diagnostic stewardship to reduce rates, healthcare expenditures and accurately identify cases of hospital-onset Clostridioides difficile infection. Infect Control Hosp Epidemiol 2021;42:51–6.
15. MacVane SH, Nolte FS. Benefits of adding a rapid PCR-based blood culture identification panel to an established antimicrobial stewardship program. J Clin Microbiol 2016;54:2455–63.
16. Wilson MR, Sample HA, Zorn KC, et al. Clinical metagenomic sequencing for diagnosis of meningitis and encephalitis. N Engl J Med 2019;380:2327–40.
17. Ransom EM, Potter RF, Dantas G, et al. Genomic prediction of antimicrobial resistance: ready or not, here it comes. Clin Chem 2020;66(10):1278–89.
18. Shea J, Halse TA, Lapierre P, et al. Comprehensive whole-genome sequencing and reporting of drug resistance profiles on clinical cases of mycobacterium tuberculosis in New York state. J Clin Microbiol 2017;55(6):1871–82.

19. Mougari F, Loiseau J, Veziris N, et al, French National Reference Center for Mycobacteria. Evaluation of the new GenoType NTM-DR kit for the molecular detection of antimicrobial resistance in non-tuberculous mycobacteria. J Antimicrob Chemother 2017;72(6):1669–77.
20. Mizusawa M, Carroll KC. Recent updates in the development of molecular assays for the rapid identification and susceptibility testing of MRSA. Expert Rev Mol Diagn 2023;23(8):679–99. PMID: 37419696.
21. Mejia-Chew C, Dubberke ER. *Clostridium difficile* control measures: current and future methods for prevention. Expert Rev Anti-infect Ther 2018;16:121–31.
22. Dominguez F, Blodget E. Community-acquired respiratory viruses. Curr Opin Organ Transplant 2019;24(4):511–4.
23. Timbrook TT, Spivak ES, Hanson KE. Current and future opportunities for rapid diagnostics in antimicrobial stewardship. Med Clin North Am 2018;102(5): 899–911.
24. Dien Bard J, McElvania E. Panels and syndromic testing in clinical microbiology. Clin Lab Med 2020;40(4):393–420.
25. Moy AC, Kimmoun A, Merkling T, et al, PCR Multiplex Study group (PMS group). Performance evaluation of a PCR panel (FilmArray® Pneumonia Plus) for detection of respiratory bacterial pathogens in respiratory specimens: a systematic review and meta-analysis. Anaesth Crit Care Pain Med 2023; 42(6):101300.
26. Vetter P, Schibler M, Herrmann JL, et al. Diagnostic challenges of central nervous system infection: extensive multiplex panels versus stepwise guided approach. Clin Microbiol Infect 2020;26(6):706–12.
27. Gupta E, Saxena J, Kumar S, et al. Fast track diagnostic tools for clinical management of sepsis: paradigm shift from conventional to advanced methods. Diagnostics 2023;13(2):277.
28. Gu W, Miller S, Chiu CY. Clinical metagenomic next-generation sequencing for pathogen detection. Annu Rev Pathol 2019 Jan 24;14:319–38.
29. Filkins LM, Bryson AL, Miller SA, et al. Navigating clinical utilization of direct-from-specimen metagenomic pathogen detection: clinical applications, limitations, and testing recommendations. Clin Chem 2020;66(11):1381–95.
30. Tran M, Smurthwaite KS, Nghiem S, et al. Auspathogen program partners. economic evaluations of whole-genome sequencing for pathogen identification in public health surveillance and health-care-associated infections: a systematic review. Lancet Microbe 2023;S2666-5247(23):00180–5.
31. Avershina E, Khezri A, Ahmad R. Clinical diagnostics of bacterial infections and their resistance to antibiotics-current state and whole genome sequencing implementation perspectives. Antibiotics (Basel). 2023;12(4):781.
32. Munnink BBO, Worp N, Nieuwenhuijse DF, et al. The next phase of SARS-CoV-2 surveillance: real-time molecular epidemiology. Nat Med 2021;27: 1518–24.
33. Meckawy R, Stuckler D, Mehta A, et al. Effectiveness of early warning systems in the detection of infectious diseases outbreaks: a systematic review. BMC Publ Health 2022;22:2216.
34. Teh R, Tee WD, Tan E, et al. Review of the role of gastrointestinal multiplex polymerase chain reaction in the management of diarrheal illness. J Gastroenterol Hepatol 2021;36:3286–97.
35. Liu J, Almeida M, Kabir F, et al. Direct detection of shigella in stool specimens by use of a metagenomic approach. J Clin Microbiol 2018;56:013744, e1417.

36. Humphries RM, Yang S, Kim S, et al. Duodenoscope-related outbreak of a carbapenem-resistant Klebsiella pneumoniae identified using advanced molecular diagnostics. Clinical Infectious Disease 2017;65:1159–66.
37. Madera S, McNeil N, Serpa PH, et al. Prolonged silent carriage, genomic virulence potential and transmission between staff and patients characterize a neonatal intensive care unit (NICU) outbreak of methicillin-resistant *Staphylococcus aureus* (MRSA). Infect Control Hosp Epidemiol 2023;44:40–6.
38. Greninger AL, Waghmare A, Adler A, et al. Rule-out outbreak: 24-hour metagenomic next-generation sequencing for characterizing respiratory virus source for infection prevention. Journal of the Pediatric Infectious Disease Society 2017;6:168–72.
39. Ramachandran PS, Ramesh A, Creswell FV, et al. Integrating central nervous system metagenomics and host response for diagnosis of tuberculosis meningitis and its mimics. Nat Commun 2022;13:1675.
40. Sichtig H, Minogue T, Yan Y, et al. FDA-ARGOS is a database with public quality-controlled reference genomes for diagnostic use and regulatory science. Nat Commun 2019;10:3313.
41. Price TK, Realegeno S, Mirasol R, et al. Validation, implementation, and clinical utility of whole genome sequence-based bacterial identification in the clinical microbiology laboratory. J Mol Diagn 2021;23:1468–77.

Printed and bound by CPI Group (UK) Ltd, Croydon, CR0 4YY

13/10/2024

01773495-0001